The Dentist:

*America's Unsung
Healthcare Hero*

In *Million Dollar Dentistry,* internationally renowned advocate for dentists Gary Kadi showed how to create thriving practices.

In *Raise Your HDL,* Gary showed dentists how to transform their personal and financial lives.

Now, in *Unsung Healthcare Hero,* Gary issues his greatest challenge of all: for dentists to step into the gap created by the collapse of traditional medicine and become a primary healthcare provider for all Americans.

MDs have lost their unique bond with patients. Due to the cataclysmic changes in medicine, MDs see patients for mere minutes, and often don't see the same patient twice.

By contrast, dentists have constant contact with their patients, ongoing relationships, and the responsibility to care for the mouth, which is where health begins.

Dentists can leverage these assets to become America's primary healthcare providers, but only if they know how, and only if they're emotionally prepared to accept this challenge.

In *Unsung Healthcare Hero,* Gary unleashes a revolutionary approach to the practice of dentistry, in which dentists step up and take the lead in healthcare.

ARE YOU READY TO BE A HEALTHCARE HERO?
Learn how…in this game-changing new book.

The Dentist:
America's Unsung Healthcare Hero

How Dentists Will Transform American Healthcare

From the Creator of The NextLevel Practice™

GARY KADI

NextLevel Practice
Scottsdale, Arizona
Manhattan, New York

The Dentist: America's Unsung Healthcare Hero

Dedicated to
the former molar mechanics,
gum gardeners, "just" assistants,
and "front desk" people
turned total healthcare heroes.

Thank you for making a profound
difference in the lives of many.
May the truth of your purpose
and dedication to total health
and wellness for all be fully realized.

CONTENTS

The economy has crashed and the world has flattened. Here's the good news: we're standing at a defining moment in time. Now is the moment to look inside our industries and our businesses. What we're doing isn't working. We're the wealthiest, unhealthiest, and in some ways the most foolish nation. What does this mean to dentists and dentistry? In this chapter, you'll find out!

The mouth is the window to total health and wellness. We've known it for years—now the world is finally catching up. Dentistry is no longer a reactionary practice or a necessary evil. It's time to reposition our industry so that it's at the forefront of total healthcare. In this chapter, I'll introduce a dramatic paradigm shift that's going to rock your world.

Over the next few years, the US will move toward centralized, paperless medical records for every patient. It's the perfect opportunity for dental teams nationwide to rebrand themselves as "dental internists." In the past, we've failed to educate patients about what going to the dentist really means. Now we've created a new vision. The dentist's office is no longer a torture chamber. It's the epicenter of total health and wellness, and the dentist is the primary healthcare provider.

ACKNOWLEDGMENTS

To my clients: Thank you for your trust and the privilege of working with you. I know it takes a lot to allow a person into one of your most valued possessions, and I do not take our relationship lightly.

To my many mentors and manuscript readers: Thank you for your time, insight, and candor, which make this book even more valuable and easier to read and understand.

To my best friend and dear wife, Judith: Thank you from the bottom of my heart for your unconditional loving support and the birth of Rome Jacob. I admire and appreciate your beauty, grace, and love. I am completely honored to be your husband.

To my son, Rome: Thank you for the true joy of being your father. You have taken me beyond my reality of love.

To my family: Thank you for instilling great values in me and for your unconditional love and support.

To my amazing team of Unsung Heroes: What a privilege to share this amazing journey together. Your dedication and courage to bust through old thinking inspires me on a very soulful level. Taking a dent out of dentistry and putting one in the world is a huge game that doesn't happen without your drive to make a profound difference in the world.

WEALTHY, UNHEALTHY, AND UNWISE

WE LIVE IN THE WEALTHIEST COUNTRY in the world. We also live in the unhealthiest.

It doesn't take an astrophysicist to look around and see what's happening in America. There's the spike in obesity and diabetes rates. The loved ones we've lost to cancer and heart disease. The general poor level of health we experience here in the richest spot on the map.

It's not like we don't know any better. For years we've been hearing about the importance of eating well and exercising regularly. We've read about it in magazines, medical journals, online—it's no longer new news. But it isn't all up to us. The insurance companies have holistic wellness in a stranglehold, and they won't be letting go anytime soon. They've turned us into a nation of fools.

Our medical system is collapsing as we speak. The financial crash of 2008 has brought about boatloads of problems. As we stand on the cusp of massive healthcare reform, there's a lot of anxiety about managed care and

1

what it means to the average citizen. Meanwhile, insurance companies continue to wreak havoc on hard-working Americans, and doctors are overworked and underpaid. In the middle of it all is you, the dentist.

If you're like most dentists, you probably feel like you're standing on the sidelines. What's all the big-picture stuff got to do with dentistry? You go to the office every morning and you drill, fill, and bill, just like any other day. Sure, maybe a few patients are delaying treatment because the economy tanked, but it's pretty much business as usual. The medical crisis is about the doctors; the healthcare crisis is about big pharma; the financial crisis is about the government. It's got nothing to do with you. Right?

Wrong.

That's what this book is all about.

What if I told you that our current crisis had everything to do with you? That you and your profession are actually the *solution* to the big-picture problems facing America? You probably wouldn't believe me, right?

That's because you have no idea what you're capable of.

You're in good company. I've spent sixteen years helping dentists develop successful practices, and I see it everywhere I go. Dentists don't think they have anything to offer the larger debate. Their patients don't really respect them, and frankly, neither does society.

There's a pervasive negative perception of dentistry today. The industry has a relatively low status within the medical profession, and hardly any patient enjoys going to the dentist's office. The work hurts; it's uncomfortable and smelly. People think of dentists as money-grubbing technicians who always want more. There's a common perception that dentists are introverted and suicidal, and the research supports it. Of twenty-two occupations examined in Washington State, dentists had a suicide rate second only to sheepherders and wool workers.

Nobody talks about it, but we all know it's true. Dentists live, work, and breathe in a fundamental lack of respect. Even accountants have more street cred than they do. People everywhere think dentists are a joke. And since no one else respects them, why should they respect themselves?

It isn't just respect that's lacking. Dentists live in a lack of everything. Lack of time, lack of money—there's never enough of anything. That's where they exist on a daily basis. "I owe, I owe, it's off to work I go," is the refrain that pounds in their heads every morning. It's not enough. They're not enough. They live in a world of scarcity and fear.

The worst part is that we all act like we don't even notice.

There's plenty of "noise" about other problems—the minutiae of any dental practice. Everybody's talking about how to fix cancelled appointments, collect money, deal with insurance headaches, and overcome the patients' unwillingness to pay. But the dentists are focusing on the trees instead of the forest. They're running around with their hair on fire, trying to plug up the holes without changing the context. You can never step back to see the bigger picture if you can't break free of the "lack of" mentality first. You don't get what you deserve in life. You get what you *think* you deserve.[1]

---

[1] For more information on how to think your way to success, check out my previous book, *Raise Your Healthy Deserve Level*.

Sad to say, most dentists don't think they deserve very much. Take a look at the story of Mark Molajockey and you'll see what I mean.

Mark was totally frustrated and depressed, like most of the dentists I've met. "I dread waking up every morning," he said. "I've been doing this for twenty-seven years. Twenty-seven freakin' years. Every Sunday night, I hear the tick-tick-tick of the bedroom clock and it's like a bomb about to go off. And sure enough, Monday morning at 6 a.m., the bomb *does* go off: I have to go into the office.

"My team is always causing problems. They don't do what I want them to do when and how I want them to do it, and they're never consistent. I can't pay my bills. No matter how hard I work, I feel like I can't get ahead of myself. I've got mountains of debt and no retirement fund to speak of. And I'm completely under-performing. I know I am.

"But here's the thing: I *like* doing dentistry. I actually enjoy what I do. It's all the other stuff that gets to me. I sedate my patients, but sometimes I wish I could sedate my team so I wouldn't have to deal with them, either! I'm so tired of having to oversee everything. I feel locked to the chair."

Mark was frustrated in his relationships to his patients, too. No matter how much he gave, his patients saw him as the bad guy. They didn't want to show up and they didn't want to pay him when they did. Every time he walked into a room, he felt unwanted and unappreciated. He worked hard to get his patients healthy and well and all they had to say was "How much will it hurt?" and "How much will it cost?"

He was miserable in the office, but he was just as miserable out of it. Everywhere he went, Mark encountered the unspoken hierarchy that says dentists aren't real doctors. Even at his own club he got the cold shoulder from neurologists and plastic surgeons. They never said it, but they didn't have to—it was all over their faces. They thought of Mark as "just a dentist," a Joe Shmoe who didn't know how the whole body worked the way they did. Sure, he was a nice guy, but he wasn't really a *doctor*.

This exacerbated Mark's own feelings of insecurity. He had chosen dentistry as his profession when he didn't get into any of his top choices for med school. To his surprise, he ended up liking the work. He was also drawn to the quality of life that dentistry promised—not having to be on call, ski trips on the weekends. But now, more than thirty years later, he felt frustrated and inadequate, and the lifestyle was a long way from what he'd imagined in dental school. Everyone considered him a dentist by default, and Mark thought of himself that way, too.

Then there was Mark's team. Dr. Molajockey thought *he* had it bad, but he had no idea what was going on in the rest of the office. Karen, his office manager, was up to her ears in phone calls and paperwork, and there never seemed to be enough hours in the day to get it all done. She wanted to wring the necks of the rest of the office staff who never seemed to be interested in doing anything besides checking their Facebook accounts. The phone was constantly ringing and the patient files were piling up, and there were her assistants, sneaking text messages to their friends when they thought she wasn't looking.

The dental hygienists and assistants were working hard, but they felt like they were never heard or understood. Mark thought of himself as "just a dentist," and their patients thought of them as "cleaning ladies" and "just assistants." They felt like no matter what they did, they couldn't make a difference. They wanted to make more money and take on more responsibilities, but they didn't know how. The patients didn't listen to them, either, and they ended up feeling discouraged.

Pam, the team leader, was the most discouraged of all. She felt like she had some good ideas for how to make the office run more smoothly, but she couldn't get them executed because nobody was on the same page. She had a new baby at home and was barely getting any sleep at night, but she was there every morning before anyone else. How did Mark reward her for her dedication? By grumbling about outstanding payments and patient no-shows.

Pam had a lot of energy, but Mark was constantly shutting her down. No matter how well she did and how much patients appreciated her positive attitude, he'd find something wrong with the way she did things. She felt like she was carrying the load and getting no respect for it. In fact she was starting to think about getting a position in another practice. Her job was rapidly turning into a dead end.

There were times when Mark was vaguely aware of his behavior toward his team. He didn't like that he was always telling people what to do, but he didn't feel like he had any other choice. Of course, even when people followed his instructions, he rarely got the result he was looking for.

What Mark didn't know was that he was playing by the rules of an outdated paradigm. He was reading from an old script and demanding that his team do the same. When things didn't go the way he wanted them to, he ended up taking out his negativity on his team. He perceived himself as nothing more than a molar jockey, and they were the molar jockey's assistants. Instead of swinging for the fences, he was sitting on the bench.

Things weren't going all that well in Mark's personal life, either. He used to have a decent stock portfolio, but thanks to the recession, it was ancient history. A few years back, Mark had borrowed money from his practice to get himself a sports car, which only plunged them into more debt. He'd pulled the same trick to buy his wife's dream home, and now they were looking at taking out a second mortgage and shrinking their lifestyle to make it all work. His wife wasn't exactly happy about that. Neither were his kids. They thought they were all entitled to Lexus SUVs the day they turned sixteen.

To distract himself from the brewing problems at home, Mark was starting to pay more attention to Amber, a new hygienist at the office. Amber was pretty and young, and she seemed responsive to his casual flirtations. Every smile she sent in his direction did wonders for Mark's chronically low self-esteem. Sometimes he fantasized about chucking his Blackberry in a dumpster and surprising Amber with one-way tickets to Maui. He knew it was crazy, but after Amber brushed up against him twice in one day, he was starting to give it serious thought.

Give Mark a few more killer Monday mornings, and his whole life is going to veer rapidly off track.

Unfortunately, Mark's story is far from unique. His problems hit close to home for most of the dentists I know. Everywhere they go in their underwear, they're dealing with the same lack of respect—the lack of respect that others show their profession, and the lack of respect they have for themselves. They live in constant doubt and uncertainty, and it shows up in their jobs and in their relationships. In my personal work with dentists, I've noticed that 70-80 percent have been divorced at least once. That's a lot higher than the 50 percent divorce rate for the general public.

So this is the world you live in. This is the prestigious world of dentistry, undressed. This is what you've gotten yourself into.

And you're about to thank your lucky stars that you did.

I'm going to show you why your self-esteem should be off the charts. I'm going to reveal why you—yes, you—are poised to be America's Unsung Healthcare Hero. Because dentistry—yes, dentistry—is going to save the day.

We're standing at a defining moment in our nation's history. Not only for the future of the world, but for the future of dentistry. We've come to a precipice of unprecedented opportunity. Dentists suddenly have what they never expected: a chance to reposition the public's perception of dentistry, and by doing so, to catapult themselves into the forefront of the fight to make America wealthy, healthy, and wise.

The economic crisis has flattened everything in our world, forcing us to look inside our businesses and industries. Imagine an Etch-a-Sketch. It's covered in scrawls and scribbles, but when you shake it out, you've got a blank canvas with which to reinvent. Because of the crash, everyone is on a level playing field, allowing us to recreate the future however we want. In our current defining moment, we've set a course for recalibration. Now all we need is someone to steer the ship.

Of course, the problem with most defining moments is that you don't know about them until they've already passed you by. At that point, all you can do is look back on them and go "woulda, coulda, shoulda." I can't tell you how many times I've kicked myself for not investing in downtown San Diego in the early 90s. Back then, there *was* no downtown, and I was just about the only person living in an apartment in the area. Now, thanks to successful urban renewal projects, it's one of the newest, hottest, and most dynamic metropolitan areas in the country.

The reason I'm writing this book is so that you won't look back on this defining moment and say "woulda, coulda, shoulda." Now is the time that you should, you could, and you *can*. I'm speaking the future in the present.

Right now, we have all the ingredients to synthesize a quantum leap in people's relationship to dentistry. Gone are the days of being sidelined and ridiculed, disrespected and scorned. Dentists are gum gardeners and molar jockeys no longer; they're the face of the revolution. If dentists are the meek, then they're about to inherit the earth.

In this new future we're about to create, *you* are going to take the lead in healthcare. That's right: the solution to our country's lack of overall health and wisdom lies in dentists and dental teams.

President Obama has recently announced his plan to cut government spending by $2 trillion over the next ten years. One way they're cutting costs is by centralizing medical records. By 2014, everything has to be digital, which will trim administrative costs substantially. While there's an ongoing debate about whether or not that's a good thing, it's the biggest gift to dentistry that we ever could have imagined. The new system will allow practitioners to tap into this centralized medical record, which will enable them to treat every patient accurately. For our purposes, "practitioner" means you.

The mouth is the gateway to total health and wellness. We've known it for years; now the scientific literature is finally catching up to us. Inflammation in the mouth is a key indicator for inflammation in the vital organs. As you know, most people don't want to deal with getting a total physical—it's a pain in the neck. Yet, most people find a way to make it to the dentist's office once or twice a year for a teeth cleaning and checkup.

Do you see where I'm going? If you are able to reinvent your practice so that it focuses on *total* health and wellness, you're going to be repositioned ahead of medical doctors. They'll be eating your dust and you will be sending patients *to them* for their specialty of care.

Because of what's happening in this country, doctors are in a kind of free fall. They're working more hours, making less money, and experiencing a lot more stress. The insurance companies have essentially taken over medicine. As a result, our entire healthcare system has been commandeered by people sitting in buildings who have no medical expertise whatsoever. That's where the "unwise" part of our predicament comes in.

Medicine is locked into a continuing downward spiral, and it's only going to get worse from here on out. The good news is, it hasn't happened in dentistry, and we can learn from their mistakes. In managed care, patients don't see the same doctor every time, let alone year after year. This has resulted in very few places where people can go to learn how to get and stay healthy, rather than suffering through a flawed system once they're already sick.

But patients always see the same dentist. They come to the same office, year after year, albeit begrudgingly. That means we now have the opportunity to educate patients, teaching them why it's important to invest beyond insurance. It's up to us to design dentistry to stay one step ahead and never fall into the same mess. It starts by shifting our focus within our practices.

Sadly, the majority of dentists focus on the hard tissue and neglect the soft, but when it comes to envisioning a whole treatment philosophy, the gums are money. What we're going to teach people is that a trip to the dentist's office is like getting a physical of the mouth. And the mouth is a key indicator of what's wrong with the whole body.

Just picture it. All the basic tests you run—blood tests, saliva scanning, checking the gums—provide invaluable information about each patient's health. Up to now, you've analyzed that data solely in regards to the state of your patient's teeth, but combined with access to the centralized medical record, these standardized tests can mean the difference between sickness and health, death and life. Your patients can be diagnosed with pre-cancer, pre-diabetes, and a host of other diseases, in *your* chair. You are the one with the power to usher each patient into whole and lasting health.

This doesn't just mean exponential growth and revenue for your practice. It means transforming our whole industry by putting us ahead of traditional medicine. People are already coming into your office annually or biannually; you can become the one-stop shop for pre-diagnosing their health needs. The research linking disease to what's going on in the mouth is irrefutable. Heart disease, cancer, and even erectile dysfunction shows up in the gums!

In light of all the evidence, we can safely say that the world no longer needs the kind of dentist who has served loyally for so many years. What the world needs is something new, something bold, something infinitely more powerful. We call it the "dental internist."

We coined a new term because it signifies an entirely new mindset. Dental internists are set to reposition the future of dentistry. It's not just a term; it's a category. Dental internists include not just the dentist, but everyone on the team. This new branding informs everyone with whom we interact, whether it's the patients who come through our doors or the MDs who make snide comments at cocktail parties. Dental internists will take a brand new approach, restructuring dental practices so that they're equal to, if not *better than*, traditional practices of medicine. In this new world, it's the dental internist who is responsible for getting patients totally healthy and well.

It goes without saying that we're taking the paradigm of dentistry and turning it on its head. The divorced, downtrodden, depressed dentist is a thing of the past. The dental internist, on the other hand, is all-powerful. Their team, their colleagues, and their families recognize them as the fearless leaders of a new movement. Dentistry is no longer the ugly stepchild of medicine. It's medicine's partner.

The face of medicine has changed. Whereas it used to be focused more on holistic care of each patient through his or her lifetime, doctors are now more likely to toss out a prescription without really getting to the source of the problem. Medicine has become reactive, not proactive. Doctors have relinquished their position as caretakers, leaving insurance companies to pick up the tab. Insurance is now dictating the medical establishment, and, as we all know, they're doing a pretty bad job.

Because of how medicine has defaulted over the years, it's created a gaping opening—a vacuum of opportunity. It's like the organic movement. Ten years ago, none of us knew what "organic" meant. But as more and more information was available about eating healthily, a vacuum was created as people started seeking out organic food. Whole Foods was there to fill that need. The company rose to national prominence as a result.

Dentistry is perfectly positioned to step right into the void that the collapse of medicine has created. The new generation of dental internists is the perfect fit. We are the ones.

Unless, of course, another genre of medicine steps ahead of us.

The opening is wide, and it demands to be filled, but if we don't seize the opportunity, someone else will. Another group of practitioners will step into the limelight. What could turn out to be the defining moment of our existence will pass us by.

It's happened before and it can happen again. I'll give you an example. In baseball legend Dave Winfield's book, *Dropping the Ball,* he talks about his battle to get Major League Baseball to take on the concept of childhood obesity as a central issue. Because baseball skews older, they needed something to hang onto the kids. Childhood obesity was the perfect tie-in.

But baseball passed on the opportunity. They hemmed and hawed and wouldn't do it. No matter how much Dave pushed, they couldn't be convinced.

And then, First Lady Michelle Obama announced her *Let's Move!* campaign to combat the epidemic of childhood obesity. Who will she be teaming with in her efforts to educate, mobilize, and empower the citizens of the United States? Major League Soccer.

Childhood obesity has now been launched into the forefront of civic policy. It would have been an incredible opportunity for baseball, pumping new life, energy, and purpose into major and minor league baseball stadiums all around the country. Now it's a White House issue, and soccer's getting all the glory while baseball is nowhere to be seen. Talk about dropping the ball!

The same thing is true for us, right here, right now. If it's not the dental internists who will become the new leader in healthcare, it will be someone else. Maybe it will be the chiropractors. Or the naturopaths. What's certain is that it will be the first group who gets their act together, who has the self-esteem to stand up and say, "What we have is so vitally important that it can transform the world." Let's take the "dent" out of dentistry and make a dent in the world.

In this book, I'm going to show you why you're right for the job.

The medical system has collapsed, and people are suffering. They are crying out for a new and better way. Dentistry is on the edge of a defining moment—a historic moment for both our world and our industry. In the chapters that follow, I'm going to lay out for you how to take advantage of this opportunity to change everything—your practice, your relationships, your life. In so doing, you're going to change the world.

So step up to the plate. You're not in the dugout anymore. The time has come for you to prove your worth, and the time is now. Your new position as a world leader will translate into more respect, better care, and greater returns, but only if you own up to who you are and what you have to offer the world.

If you're not ready for the adventure of a lifetime, then have a nice day drilling, filling, and billing.

But if you *are* ready, read on.

Chapter 1 — Takeaways

> ❯ We're the wealthiest, unhealthiest, and in some ways, the most foolish nation in the world.

> ❯ Traditional medicine is no longer working and medical doctors are in free fall. It's time to make a change.

> ❯ Dentists suffer from low self-esteem and lack of respect. They're in survival mode, operating out of scarcity and fear.

> ❯ Because of the economic crisis, things have been flattened. Now is the perfect time to reevaluate, recalibrate, and reposition ourselves as leaders in healthcare.

> ❯ Dentists have the capacity to revolutionize the medical profession, becoming the primary caregiver for millions of Americans.

> ❯ It's time to shift your practice and your mindset away from being a dentist and toward being a dental internist.

> ❯ You and your profession have the power to change the world.

THE RUBBER DAM
HITS THE DENTAL ROAD

I F YOU'RE AS OLD AS I AM and you're a sports fan, you probably remember the "Miracle on Ice." Let me take you back there for a moment…

It was the 1980 Winter Olympics at Lake Placid, New York. The Soviets were the world champions in hockey, having medaled every year since 1963. The US men's team, coached by Herb Brooks, was made up of amateur and collegiate players. Of the twenty guys on the roster, only one had played at the Olympic level. It didn't look good for the good ol' US.

In the semifinal game with the Soviets (most people think it was the finals!), we fell behind early, but the first period ended in a 2-2 tie. In the second period, tensions mounted as the Soviets dominated play, outshooting the Americans 12-2 but scoring only once. After two periods, the Soviet Union led 3-2.

Then, something incredible happened. In the third period, Team USA scored two goals, catapulting them to

4-3, their first lead of the game with only ten minutes left on the clock.

The Soviets fought back and the final minutes of the game were intense. With less than twenty seconds remaining, the crowd began a countdown. That's when ABC sportscaster Al Michaels picked up the countdown on his broadcast and delivered his famous call:

"Eleven seconds, you've got ten seconds, the countdown going on right now! Morrow, up to Silk...five seconds in the game...Do you believe in miracles?...YES!"

And the US took home the gold.

The International Ice Hockey Federation chose the Miracle on Ice as the number one international hockey story of the century. It's the classic tale of triumph: the underdogs become the champions. The US team had no aspirations and no expectations; nobody thought they were going to be the gold medal winners in the Olympics. Yet, they were.

Now let me ask *you* a question.

Do *you* believe in miracles?

What I'm about to share with you is going to seem pretty miraculous. After a lifetime of being diminished and demeaned for your profession, why wouldn't it? But all that's about to change.

In this chapter, I'm going to show you how the MDs are like the Soviets, and you're like the US 1980 men's hockey team. You, too, can go from nowhere to gold medal status. It begins not in the mouth of the Russians' goal, but in the mouth of your patients.

Why the mouth?

The mouth is the window to total health and wellness.

We breathe through our mouths. We communicate through our mouths. We eat through our mouths. The mouth is where food gets chewed up and our body begins digesting it; it's where oxygen goes in and carbon dioxide comes out. Except in the case of an injection, most things that enter the body come through the mouth.

Hey, we kiss with our mouths!

Because the mouth is so important, there's a lot that can go wrong. If you don't tend to the mouth, bacteria can manifest there and travel through the bloodstream, affecting the other organs. This can have a serious effect on how the rest of the body functions. For example, C-reactive proteins in your blood rise when there's inflammation in your gums. Inflamed soft tissue can indicate all sorts of problems.

Your mouth is a key indicator of wellness, reflecting what's going on in the rest of your body. If you're healthy, your mouth will look good. If you're unhealthy, your mouth will bear the evidence.

Dentists know all this. When I stand up at a seminar and say that the mouth is the gateway to health, nobody disagrees. I'm putting words to the music that's already in their heads. But there's a departure between knowledge and action. They may *know* how important the mouth is to total wellness, but their focus is elsewhere. Their focus is on survival—just closing enough cases to meet payroll, pay the rent, and pay down their American Express cards. (Are you with me yet?)

The dental industry has bamboozled a lot of well-intentioned people. From the outside, being a dentist looks really good: money, freedom, all the perks. But what dentists don't realize is that they have to go beyond the chairside work to actually run a business. That's when the reality of fear, scarcity, and survival sets in.

What this means is that most dentists pool all their time and attention into one area: the hard tissue. It's all about the teeth. The mindset of dentistry has become, "My patients only have a finite amount of money, so I better just diagnose the hard tissue." They end up practically ignoring the soft tissue, when it's the soft tissue that's an integral part of oral systemic health. This is where the rubber hits the road. Or, as we like to say in the industry, where the rubber dam hits the dental road.

The soft tissue is chronically under-diagnosed in dentistry today. Even when there's proof that something may be wrong, dentists tend to look the other way. Consider the occurrence of bleeding. Bleeding of the gums is not acceptable. Your scalp doesn't bleed when you brush your hair! But most offices allow for bleeding, telling the patient it's not a problem. The patient hears this, believes it, and doesn't take action. For dentistry to rise to the leading edge of healthcare, we've got to start recognizing bleeding as a tangible indicator that total wellness has yet to be achieved.

According to the research, 75 percent of adults have some form of periodontal disease, *aka* inflammation of the gums. Those inflamed gums indicate that there's inflammation elsewhere in the body. It all boils down to inflammation. Studies have shown that patients with inflammation in the mouth have a 62 percent increase of pancreatic cancer and a 92 percent increase of diabetes. There's also a high correlation between inflammation and heart disease. What's going on in the soft tissue is a major indicator of overall health.

It's the soft tissue that tells the story of what's going on elsewhere in the patient's body. So if we want to reposition dentists as the primary healthcare providers in America, it's time we develop a hard focus on the soft areas.

Doing so requires a seismic shift. When I work with dentists, I always ask, "What's the first question you ask a returning patient?" The way they answer that question lets me know where their focus is.

If they say, "Are you having any problems?", it means they're a "fixer." The scope of their dental work begins and ends with fixing problems; they pay very little attention to preventative care.

If they say, "Does anything hurt you?", it means they're pain relievers. The scope of these practices is limited to finding and alleviating pain.

If a dentist asks, "What brings you into the office today?", it's more of an open-ended question. That's a step in the right direction, but it's still not as good as it could be. Chances are, people either come to a dentist to get pain relief or because it's raining really hard outside and they can't get a cab to their MD's office.

At NextLevel Practice, we teach dentists to broaden the focus of their attention by significantly widening their scope. The absolute best question to ask a patient is: "How's your overall health?"

Because it's such an unusual question to hear in a dental office, the patient may very well ask, "Why are you asking me that?"

This gives the dentist the perfect opportunity to say, "Well, let me explain. Here in our practice, we take on your total health. What happens in your mouth is a gateway to wellness, in your body, mind, and soul."

The patient is intrigued and impressed. In one succinct statement, the dentist has now launched himself into the game of total health.

The dentist is a newcomer to this game. There are already a lot of players out on the ice—the GPs, the MDs, the insurance companies who claim to care about getting people well when really they make their money keeping people sick. Then, of course, you have to contend with the perceptions of the general public. If you tell people the mouth is the gateway to total health, they're probably going to use their mouth to laugh in your face. Who cares about the mouth?

It's sad but true. The mouth is the Rodney Dangerfield of the body; it doesn't get any respect. Ever wondered why cardiovascular surgeons are the most respected and highest paid doctors in medicine? Or why the expression goes, "It's not brain surgery!", when something's easy, instead of, "It's not dentistry!"? It's because the heart and the brain get all the attention. People vote with their dollars and their respect, and those two areas are the ones that get it.

I'm not saying that the heart and brain aren't important. If your brain's not working you can't think, and if your heart's not working you can't live. But you generally have to be sick in a lot of other ways before you develop brain or heart illness. Once any illness or disease gets to the level of interfering with your brain activity or stopping your heartbeat, of course, it's too late. So I'm talking about the mouth as the *indicator* of serious problems. I'm talking about taking preventative measures, and using dentistry to do it.

In Western society, we want tangible, direct connections, and we want them *now*. The mindset of human beings is geared primarily toward survival. If somebody finds out they have a brain tumor, they schedule surgery. If somebody has a heart attack, they get a stent put in. But if someone has inflammation of the mouth, they're less likely to draw a parallel between their sore gums and what's happening in the rest of their body. There's no urgency, no tangibility. You can live with cavities, but you can't live with a bad heart.

By the way, dentists aren't the only ones who suffer from this mindset. It's one of the main problems facing chiropractors. Most people are vaguely aware that subluxations affect the nervous system, but they're too far removed from direct hits.

That's why it's imperative that we shift the paradigm. Long before the brain tumor or the heart attack reveals itself, dentists have the opportunity to *recognize and diagnose sickness and disease.* Everything that goes on in the body—how the brain is fed through the bloodstream, the pumping of the heart—can be sourced from what goes through the mouth and how it functions.

At this point you may be saying, "Gary, if you think that dentists are going to get the same respect as heart surgeons and brain surgeons, you're crazy. It's totally impossible."

You're right—it's *been* totally impossible. Right up until this moment.

We have a very short window of opportunity to change the perception of dentists in America and beyond. The world has been flattened because of the financial crash, and the way people are spending their money is changing. We're beginning to notice the following trend. People are investing less in luxury items to look good on the outside, and more on things to keep them alive and well. If we can show people that a trip to the dentist is the way to do it, we'll have the market cornered.

There are several reasons for this shift. The baby boomer generation is getting older and their thinking has changed. A decade ago there was a rise in tummy tucks and face lifts because they wanted to look younger; today they want to live longer. The boomers are a key demographic. Even though their IRAs have been affected by the economic crash, they're spending money on practical things to keep them alive longer—e.g., organic foods, acupuncture, yoga classes, fish oil. On paper they've lost money, but they still have plenty of cash, in part due to the inheritances that many of them have received. These people are willing to pay more for preventative health than ever before, and now that healthcare is in total disarray, people don't know where to turn. They're searching for answers, and their money is going to go to the first group that supplies them.

As we stand on the brink of a centralized medical history, the barriers are crumbling. It's like we're about to bust down the Berlin Wall between dentistry and medicine. When a patient sees that you are operating on the same plane as her GP, she's going to take note. You, her dentist, are contributing to the same medical history form that her doctor contributes to. This gives a subtle message to the patient that, "Hey, this guy is just as valuable as my MD."

These conversations may be unspoken, but a new mindset doesn't need to be shouted to be understood. The US is essentially saying, "Dentistry matters." If they didn't think that dentists had anything valuable to contribute, then they wouldn't let them plug into the centralized record. The dialogue that's being created through action has already begun changing popular perceptions of dentistry.

If we can highlight that change in each of our practices, then we'll eventually reach a tipping point where there's a nationwide shift. Suddenly, people will realize that dentistry matters. Sure, their doctors are still important. But a trip to the dentist is going to be the hot new thing in healthcare that no one can afford to go without.

In Al and Laura Ries's brilliant book, *The 22 Immutable Laws of Branding*, they talk about how there's only one top brand in every business category. You know what they are—Kleenex in tissues, Tylenol in over-the-counter pain relief. In some cases the brand names have become synonymous with the item itself, like Band-Aids or Jell-O. Once you've achieved the number one position, it's hard to lose your spot.

According to their research, "A widely publicized study of twenty-five leading brands in twenty-five different product categories in the year 1923 showed that twenty of the same twenty-five brands are still the leaders in their categories today. In seventy-five years, only five brands lost their leadership."

We all know who the top dogs in medicine are. MDs are the number one brand, and for good reason: doctors save lives. It's been that way forever. They saved my dad's life and they saved mine; I'm sure they've saved the lives of your friends and family members, too. I've got no problem with doctors—in fact I'm very grateful to them for all their amazing work.

The problem comes when that true statement— "Doctors save lives"—becomes an automatic filter. It dictates the inner monologue all dentists have playing on repeat. Doctors save lives; dentists, on the other hand, are costly, suicidal, and unnecessary. Doctors are vital members of society; dentists have been at the bottom of the totem pole.

But now that the playing field has been leveled, the filters have been lowered. Consumers are starting to realize that what they've been doing—spending a lot of money on doctors and prescriptions—is not fixing the problem. It's actually exacerbating it. Money is the driving force of healthcare. The drug companies have made a killing on America's sickness and disease; the more symptoms that patients manifest, the more money in the bank. If Americans start getting healthy, big pharma will no longer be needed.

What's happening in the prescription drug arena is the stuff nightmares are made of. For example, did you know that the Federal Drug Administration has a fast track for drugs? If you pay the FDA $250,000, you can have your drugs on the market in six months instead of the standard two to three years—no long-term clinical testing required. The government is prostituting itself to big pharma, which just reinforces the power of the doctors since they're the ones who do the prescribing. Even long-term tests are only run for a year or two. Who knows what's going to happen five or ten years down the line if you keep taking a drug? Your guess is as good as mine.

Doctors are at the mercy of the system, locked in to a continuing downward spiral, but what's bad for them is great for you. Because people are seeing that the old system no longer works, they're looking for new solutions to old problems, and you're the one who's got the answers. The catalyst for pioneering total health and wellness resides in your chair. Together, we're going to knock off medicine as the number one healthcare brand.

Branding is perceived in the minds of the consumer. It's all perception. You can't blame them—people do the best they can with the awareness they have. If their only awareness is that medicine is the place to go, then that's where they're going to stay, but if you do your part to raise the collective awareness, then people will begin to understand that dentistry is the place to go. The statistics will change, and medicine will be one of those five in twenty-five brands that got knocked out of the top spot.

It's not only up to the dentist. The dental assistants play their part as well. The most influential person on a dental team is the assistant—they have the most one-on-one interactions with patients and the best shot at earning their trust. Unfortunately, many assistants perceive their jobs as a one-way street to nowhere. But in our work with dental practices across the country, we work closely with assistants to enable to them to fully express their unique gifts and talents. As a result, it transforms how people perceive dentistry, because the patient no longer feels that the assistant is just trying to sell them something. That's the beauty of the movement toward systemic oral health: it starts at a grassroots level.

Imagine the following scenario.

You're no longer bumping into rocks, cleaning teeth and filling cavities day in and day out. Your focus has shifted from the hard tissue to include the soft, and the floodgates have burst open. You're finally paying attention to what you've always known—the mouth is the window to total health and wellness. You're a dental internist through and through.

Your role in the larger scheme of healthcare is no longer inconsequential. As a matter of fact, you're hugely influential in terms of getting people healthy and securing the treatment they need. You're no longer focused on survival and just getting through the day. Instead, every moment with a patient is an opportunity to educate, heal, and empower. The mouth isn't just a site for cavities and bad breath; it's a key indicator. Combined with the centralized medical record, it gives essential clues and evidence for what's going on in the rest of the body.

Finally, after years of drudgery, you're doing the kind of dentistry you want to do—helping people live and be well. Instead of slaving for your practice, your practice is working for you. This allows you to slow down, take good care of your patients, and thoroughly educate them through your hygiene department. Your patients respect and believe you; they know that your office is the starting point for their journey to whole health.

Right now this movement is catching on like wildfire. We will reach the tipping point when dentists have become the most trusted healthcare practitioners of all healthcare practitioners. You and your profession will have essentially gone from busking on the side of the road to being the rock stars of healthcare.

Sounds pretty good, right? So how do you make it happen?

It starts in your office.

What happens in your office that helps bring on this revolution is revealed in the next chapter. Once you discover that guidance…you'll believe in miracles, too.

Chapter 2 — Takeaways

> The mouth is the window to total health and wellness.

> The soft tissue is where the rubber dam hits the dental road. It's the key indicator in oral systemic health.

> Long before brain and heart problems manifest, dentists have the opportunity to *recognize and diagnose sickness and disease.*

> The baby boomer generation is more interested in preventative care than ever before. They're willing to make a big investment, and they've got the funds to do it.

> The centralized medical record is going to break down the Berlin Wall between dentistry and medicine.

> Dentists have the potential to become the primary healthcare practitioners in America, knocking MDs out of the top spot.

> Nationwide change starts at a grassroots level. It begins with you.

CHAPTER 3

THE MOVEMENT BEGINS, ONE PRACTICE AT A TIME

ORE THAN TWO HUNDRED YEARS AGO, thirty-four
of our nation's forefathers gathered around a table to
sign the Declaration of Independence. Forged by Thomas
Jefferson and breathed into being by the US Congress, the
document announced our independence from England
and mapped out the future of our great country.

One year ago, thirty-four men and women gathered
around a different table, this one in Cancun, Mexico. The
document we crafted was also a declaration, one that not
only envisioned a future for our great country, but a future
for our great industry as well.

That's right. I'm talking about dentistry.

It may sound crazy to compare dentistry to the
Declaration of Independence, but we're talking about a
movement that's already happening and that we believe
will continue to take the nation by storm. We're talking
about a complete and total reinvention of our relationship
to dentistry, so that it is the dentists in the United States

who answer the call to healthcare reform and pioneer wellness nationwide. You, the dentist and dental teams, are going to be the new American heroes. Now how's that for a declaration?

At our annual event in Cancun, I stood at a whiteboard and asked thirty-four powerful people, including my team, other dentists, and their spouses or significant others, to join me in an exercise. I asked them to call out everything that had been associated with dentistry up to this point. They had no trouble tossing out words—expensive, unnecessary, painful, smelly, a rip-off. You can probably come up with your own list of all the pejorative terms and put-downs. It ain't pretty.

Then we flipped the page and did what we call a "blank slate" exercise. We started speaking about dentistry in the twenty-first century and the future of our industry. The dentists started throwing out new words, new ideas—what the field of dentistry really is today, and everything it can be.

The exciting thing about this movement is that it already exists. We're not starting from scratch; we are just picking up on the momentum that's already there. Dentists and dental teams across the country are beginning to move out of the old paradigm to become *pioneers of total health and wellness for all.* It won't be long before the movement spreads like wildfire. It happens one practice at a time.

There are really two movements going on at the same time. Pioneering total health and wellness is the second movement. The first movement paves the way for it, because it begins in your office and expands outwards. I'm talking about the DDS movement, and I don't mean Doctor of

Dental Surgery. I'm talking about *Dentists Deserve Success*. The two movements have to go in lockstep with one another to come to fruition. And it all starts with you. In order for us to reinvent dentistry, we've got to uplevel the mindset of the dentist. Most practices today are operating at 50 percent. Why? Because an insidious negative mindset has put an unspoken restriction in place. The dentist and the entire team are functioning at half capacity because in their mind, they don't deserve any better. For many this is a blindspot.

I can't tell you how many dentists I've talked to who sell themselves short. "I'm just one little dentist from a small town in Kansas," they say. "What can *I* do? I can't make a difference in my own office, let alone a nationwide movement for the whole industry."

You're right—with that attitude, you can't. That's why we've designed a three-year program to help every dentist move toward bigger and better. The DDS program will revolutionize your practice in ways you never imagined. In this chapter, I'm going to share the basic tenets of that program, going through it step-by-step so you can achieve the same success that hundreds of other dentists have enjoyed. This, in turn, will allow you to participate in this movement, should you choose.

When I first got into this business, I was a consultant— slick suit, briefcase, the whole shebang. I rapidly found out that dentists are dealing with a severe case of consultant fatigue. Consultants talk about how to fix symptoms, and I was no different. I breezed in, dealt with symptoms, and told people what to do. And you know what? It only worked to a point and most often wasn't sustainable.

There are many great dental consultants who have elevated many practices. I was so intrigued as to why some dentists were searching for the next consult before they were finished with the one they had. It indicated that consulting wasn't satisfying the source. I kept inquiring deeper. "Maybe," I thought, "we don't have a finger on the pulse of what's really going on." When I realized this, I understood that we needed to go beneath the surface and get to the bottom of why things weren't happening for the ever-searching dentist. What do they really want that they are not getting? Then we could find a way to eliminate the reoccurring issues, so that dentists were no longer on the treadmill of broken and cancelled appointments and accounts receivable.

Instead of looking at the symptoms, we focus our attention on what's causing them. When you knock out the problems at the source, you can put your attention on the stuff that matters: doing the type of dentistry you want to do, focusing on customer service, and being outcome-based instead of activity-based. This is an educational curriculum, not consulting.

In Year One, we install a new methodology. We essentially map out a new and improved future for how the practice will run. The old model was, "Throw up a shingle, get your roller skates on, and giddyup." But in today's world, we don't recommend that you fly by the seat of your pants. Instead, we put an infrastructure in place to double the size of the practice in twelve months.

It may sound impossible, but I've seen it happen for a countless number of dentists in practices all over the United States. It's about making a fundamental shift from working harder to working smarter. That's what Year One is all about. It's not just in the workplace; the results show up at home as well. Dentists and team members experience a breakthrough in their relationship to time, money, and the people in their lives, whether it's friends, family, or their colleagues. Once you put people development and business development in place, everything in your life will expand.

You may be saying, "Yeah, but..." I've worked with plenty of "Yeah but"s over the last few decades. Maybe you've worked with a consultant before and had less-than-stellar results, or your team didn't buy into it. What's different about our approach is its simplicity. One of the things my grandfather taught me was how to take something complex and simplify it. That's what I do when I work with dentists. Information without action has no value, so our attention is on the art and science of implementing actual change.

What I found in working with dentists is that everything is so complex. It's like the professors in dental school—they take complex things and instead of simplifying them, they make them more complex. We do the opposite. We simplify the art of running a practice, which creates huge value for you. In today's busy world, nobody wants more things to do. They want *fewer* items on the To Do list. So I set out to create something very simple. It's a method I call "radical common sense."

I took the radical common sense approach to dentistry. I went to dental offices around the country and got the truth from patients and team members. I discovered that dentists, much like I did as a consultant, dealt primarily with symptoms and not the truth. They were basically dealing with a moving target. So I analyzed what people were doing and how they were working, and I worked backward from there to create a radical common sense solution, which I outline in detail in my first book, *Million Dollar Dentistry*.

The Year One curriculum teaches several basic keys to practice development. It teaches dental teams how to create a new patient for life and to retain existing patients once they've got them. The average retention in practices is about 40 percent when I begin working with them. Not so hot!

I also work with dentists and dental teams to create a fundamental paradigm shift, moving away from the idea that "most people can't afford dentistry." This isn't the truth. People actually *can* afford things they really want; the problem is that we haven't done a good job of showing them *why* they want it. When was the last time you bought something you didn't think you needed that was going to cost you thousands of dollars, would probably hurt, and was going to take time out of your day? When I asked this at a live event someone yelled out, "CONSULTING!" Perfect!

At the core of Year One methodology is the five-step process that dentists have implemented across the country. This process has transformed countless dental practices, and it can transform yours, too.

STEP 1 – The Infrastructure

We begin by working backward. I have dentists look at where they want to end up, and from there we do a little reverse-engineering. In other words, we put an infrastructure in place.

Every practice is different from the next, yours included. You've got different patients, a different mindset about treatment planning, a different team structure, different equipment, and a different dental philosophy. It's important to try and get a handle on every single nuance about a practice. Only then can we truly understand the current situation, as well as map out where you want to go.

If you ask someone where they want to go, most people don't really know. They just know they want more of something—more time, more money. That's why Step 1 is crucially important: we're actually defining, on paper, where you want to end up. We work with each person on the team to get them to define the lifestyle they ultimately want, and then we work backward to quantify it.

We ask the dentist questions like: How many hours do you want to work? What type of dentistry do you want to do? How do you want to pay your team? When do you want to have your debt paid off? What kind of retirement do you want to end up with?

Only 2 percent of dentists end up financially free at the end of their careers. Did you get that statistic? Ninety-eight percent of dentists work their whole careers and have little to nothing in the bank to show for it. How disheartening is that?

It's our goal to reverse that statistic, so that 98 percent of dentists are sitting pretty in their golden years, doing what they like to do, instead of still sitting chairside, doing what they have to do. So we'll start with the end in mind and work backward, in order to lay out a feasible infrastructure for achieving tangible success.

STEP 2 – The Plan

I have experienced that most advisors deal with symptoms by employing tactics instead of reinventing the baseline *strategy*. When we co-create a plan with the dentist in Step 2, we focus on strategy, a step-by-step plan that leverages the three ways to grow a practice: Case Acceptance, Patient Retention, and the Experience for the New Patient. We also instill the triple-win mindset where the patient, team, and dentist win, with no one left out.

This allows for the dentist and team to be responsible and accountable to the new consumer. The new consumer is different than before the financial crash. People today have a completely different mindset. They buy practical items rather than luxury items. Money may be tighter than before, but they'll pay for items that they perceive have value. You can't actually create value if you don't have the right people in the right place doing the right things with the right mindset about what they're really offering.

This is one of the fundamental paradigm shifts we initiate in a dental practice. Instead of being a torturer whose only job is to fix pain and problems, dentists begin to present to the patient what the patient truly wants: health, function, and aesthetics.

To do this, we co-create a plan with the dentist and the team based on the feedback they give us. They actually help us create the solution. They *know* what needs to happen, but there's typically a gap between knowledge and implementation. And that's where we come in.

STEP 3 – The Blank Slate

Just as we did with our thirty-four forefathers of future dentistry in Cancun, we use the blank slate exercise in our work with individual practices. The blank slate gives us the opportunity to reinvent how the future is going to go. It allows us to pull off the rearview mirror and stop letting our present be dictated by our past.

What's great about blank slating is that we're working side by side with dentists. It's their practice; we're not coming in as a third party to tell them what to do. We're raising people's awareness and having them make changes from the inside out, versus us trying to make changes from the outside in. It's the difference between change and transformation. This also happens from year to year so that quantum leaps can occur throughout your career.

STEP 4 – Getting Agreement

Step 4 is about gaining consensus on a dental team. Instead of the dentist telling her team members what to do, it's important that she hold them accountable to the agreements they made. In order to do this, they've got to understand why they're doing what they're doing.

We teach our teams to ask questions about *why* they're doing something, because now they're going to operate from a contextual standpoint. They won't be doing something simply because they're told to. When we have team members asking *how* to do things, it means they haven't bought into the system and aren't able to think on their own feet. That's the difference between *why* and *how* thinking. The sooner we can get the members of a dental team to move from how to why, the sooner there is agreement from the inside, not one that is imposed, and the practice can move forward.

STEP 5 – Implementing and Refining

You can plan, devise, and design until you're blue in the face, but until you put it out on the court, it's not going to work. In Step 5 we implement and refine the plan we've come up with, and then we measure and monitor it until it's producing the right results.

One of the benefits to our program is that we've got a strong backend. We lock people into their commitments to ensure they meet their goals. Everybody needs a coach or a trainer in their corner. For me personally, I don't like going to the gym. That's why it's important that every Tuesday and Thursday, my personal trainer shows up and ensures that I work out hard. I've got a *why* to my work—I'm building muscle for the future so I can continue to work with dentists around the country. At forty-six, I want to be around for a long time to share life with Judith and my son, Rome. I also have systems of measurements in place to mark and monitor my progress—how much I'm lifting, my target weight. Whenever I veer off track, my trainer brings me back into line.

Our default mechanism as human beings is to go to the small negative places. It's nobody's fault; it's just human nature. So to help dentists achieve measurable, *repeatable* success, we put in a coaching structure.

That doesn't mean our clients are dependent on us—far from it. As the saying goes, "Give a man a fish and you feed him for a day. Teach a man to fish and you feed him for a lifetime." We're definitely not giving fish to our clients. Instead, we teach them how to fish by empowering dentists to manage their practices and empowering dental teams to educate patients. The dental teams we work with are self-reliant entities who benefit greatly from (and appreciate) our support.

At the end of Year One, every member of a dental practice feels newly empowered and competent; they see the vision more clearly than ever before, and they're dedicated to working with one another to achieve it.

One of the key players who emerges in our model is the team leader. In the old-school paradigm, we had the office manager—the one pushing papers around in a back room. By contrast, the new-school team leaders are out there on the court, proactively supporting their teams, measuring daily primary outcomes of each team member, listening to patients, and pushing the practice forward toward the common goal: pioneering total health and wellness for everyone.

That includes the team first. This is where the integrity piece comes in. If you're going to be pioneering health and wellness out in the world, you better be living it yourself. If you're not, it doesn't mean that you're bad; it just means you have to come back to taking care of yourself first. We believe dentistry can be a catalyst in all areas of health and wellness—not just physical, but mental, emotional, and financial as well.

That's what's exciting about Year One: it sows all the seeds for a dazzling future and the ability to be a part of a powerful community dedicated to serving others. One dentist we worked with increased his collections from $50,000 to $70,000...by the second month! That's a 40 percent increase in sixty days. Imagine what you could do in 365!

Can you imagine how free you would be if cash flow worries were no longer waking you up at 4 a.m.?

But soon we began to notice something strange was happening. After dentists and dental teams experienced quantum leaps in their relationships to time, money, and people, they began to slip backwards into their old habits. Even when they were making substantially more money, they felt like they didn't deserve it.

Think about moving a tooth. Even after you do the work, the periodontal ligament wants to pull the tooth back to its original position—it feels natural that way. That's why it's important that patients wear their retainers to keep the new position of the teeth until it becomes a habit.

That's exactly how it is for you and your new lease on life and dentistry. In Year One, you've created muscles. You've realized that there's more money for you and your team, and that your patients have the money to pay you because you are providing a huge value for them. Every person who comes through your front door has an entirely different perception of you and of dentistry in general; they know why they come in to your office and why they should come back.

But if you don't continue to practice your revolution-ary new approach, you'll fall back into old habits. The same goes for all the great sports legends. Tiger Woods, Kobe Bryant, Derek Jeter—there's a reason why they go to the driving range and shoot free throws and take fielding practice over and over again, even after they've just won a game. Or a championship. If you don't practice what you learned in Year One and keep it alive and thriving, it will be just like the periodontal ligament pulling you back.

That's why during Year Two, we focus on sustainability. You've already built the new muscles for running a practice, having more money, and having more time. Now you have to learn how to *be* with it. In Year Two, we work with dentists to help them be okay with the fact that they're working fewer hours and making twice the amount of money. We want them to learn to live with all the positive changes in their lives—their team is happy, their patients are happy, their wife and kids are happy. Now it's time that they're happy, too, and that they stay that way.

For most of the dentists we work with, their whole life has been a challenge. They've become so accustomed to resistance that they end up creating more on an ongoing basis for themselves! So why not resist the need to invent resistance? There is a point where the focus goes from looking for the next set of problems to focusing on the next set of solutions. This shift opens up the doors to allowing a new level of transformation to take place.

I've seen incredible things happen with dental practices during Year Two. Everybody takes a different path. We have dentists who bring on associates. Some dentists decide to buy other practices and duplicate the process. Others are preparing to become a NextLevel Learning Center where they give away what they learned to other practitioners in their region. Then there are the dentists who are taking more free time for themselves; their "resistance" comes in the form of learning how to lead a simple and balanced life. Whatever it is, we work with the dentist to create a workable plan. They get to design their lifestyle—the lifestyle they've always wanted and dreamed about.

That's where HDL—Healthy Deserve Level—comes in. It's what inspired me to write my second book, *Raise Your Healthy Deserve Level*. If you don't believe you deserve success, then you won't be able to hold onto it once you've achieved it. In other words, a dentist's "periodontal ligament" is a low deserve level. The same thing goes for your team. If their HDL is low, they won't continue to create results and value for patients on an ongoing basis. When the HDL machine stalls, so does everything else.

Year Two is a critical year. As dentists build and strengthen their HDL muscles, they begin looking at the world through a brand new set of eyes. They start to give back to their community because they finally have the time, money, and relationships to do so. It's a powerful place to come from. The fundamental question changes from "What can I get from you?" to "What can I provide for the people around me—my team, my patients, my community?" I've seen it hundreds of times—a natural shift toward generosity, kindness, fun, freedom, and peace of mind. And the best part? They learn how to live in that kind of lifestyle on a regular basis.

The foundation laid in Year One is what gets dentists to Year Two, and the skills acquired in Year Two open the doors to Year Three. This is when you experience the world-altering opportunity to transform other practices and the industry itself. Once you revolutionize *your* life and practice, you're going to find yourself eager to take on the next step.

Year Three is about pioneering health and wellness worldwide, using dentistry as the vehicle. It isn't for everybody—some dentists and their teams are perfectly happy with their progress from Years One and Two, and that's fine. But I've seen so many dentists who are ready to take this to the mat and leave dentistry in a far better position than how they found it. It's like the scope of their purpose has expanded.

It's the most organic thing in the world. In Year One, their purpose was to make money and survive. In Year Two, they want to hold on to everything they've learned and gained. In Year Three, they say, "You know what? I want to share this with others. There's enough time, money, and relationships for everyone. Let's get this show on the road!"

It's not just dentists who have a historically low HDL. It's the entire industry! Up until now, dentistry was a major headache—make that a toothache—for the majority of the population. But once a dentist has seen her practice transformed in Years One and Two, she begins looking for ways to boost the HDL of others. Her goal shifts from creating a Healthy Deserve Level not only for her team, her patients, and her community, but for dentistry as a whole. This is where the magic happens.

When I met with the thirty-four trendsetting dental leaders in Mexico, I realized that we really are on the cusp of a movement that will change dentistry forever. The work has already begun. We're creating mutual mentoring hubs and area learning centers, because people who have already had the DDS breakthrough are bringing it to their communities.

They're also bringing it to other practitioners. Now that dentists have learned that there's no scarcity of time, money, and relationships, they want to share their newfound knowledge with other dentists who are still struggling through life with a low deserve level. The old thinking was: There aren't enough patients for everyone and competition is cutthroat. The new thinking is: Only 50 percent of the public go to their dentist on a regular basis. There are plenty of patients! Patients, money, and time are all in abundance. So why not share the wealth?

Thanks to the work we get to do every day, we are seeing amazing things happen in this industry, and it all starts in the individual practices. Practitioners enjoy being chairside more, which has a significant impact on dentist-patient relationships. They also enjoy their teams—they no longer feel like they're herding cats! They've got more space in their lives and more room in their heads. They also understand that in order to keep something, they have to give back to it. So by giving back to fellow practitioners and educating them on all that's possible, they're pouring energy and effort into the dental community on a grass-roots level, and we all know how powerful grassroots can be. Just look at Barack Obama's epic 2008 presidential campaign. It sure did work for him!

The exciting thing is that the movement is already happening. People are having breakthroughs and giving back, and the message is expanding. Our job is to continue to get it out to the masses. We can't do it alone; we've got to do it together. That includes every dentist, every vendor, every consultant, every manufacturer, every dental assistant, every hygienist, every team leader, and every front office person. Your individual practice can make a huge difference if you're connected to a larger community, and that's what this movement is all about.

Think of all the other businesses in the world. Most of them are franchises—part of a community of businesses. Dentistry is one of the only businesses left that hasn't been totally franchised (although many are trying). Dentists typically value their individuality and resist the idea of being consumed by a larger group. They think they have to go it alone. What's great about the movement I'm talking about is that it allows you to come together as a community and be part of a big movement *while still maintaining your independence.*

That's the new model in today's world. It's about plugging into the greater good for the greatest amount of people. Give, give, give. According to the law of reciprocity, it's going to come back to you. Right up until this very moment, dentists have been the little guys in their little cities, too worried about getting through the day to ever see the big picture. That's where dentistry has been, but it's not where it's going.

Modern dentistry is an exciting new frontier—a land of pioneers. The movement that's happening in and outside of America demands that dentists become pioneers and frontier people, shifting first the dentists' perception of themselves, and then standing for the public's new perception of dentistry. If you're ready to pioneer total health and wellness, great! Hop aboard.

You may be saying, "I *want* to believe you, Gary. But I don't even know where to begin." That's okay. The journey of a thousand miles begins with a single step. Simply take the first action. It could be as easy as setting up a consult room so you have a private area to educate patients. Or getting your hygienists to start using intraoral cameras. Maybe it's time to write out your purpose as a dentist and to get your dental team to write out theirs.

You might decide that now's the time to get clear on your philosophy of what a healthy mouth is and what it isn't (we call this the "healthy mouth baseline"), and to articulate it with your team and your patients. Or you might take it up a notch and go into your community to start talking about dentistry and what it really provides. I'm working with a number of dentists who are taking what they learned in Years One and Two of the program and creating learning centers in their communities so that they can share the same tools with everyone else.

You don't have to participate in our programs to join the movement. I'm giving my strategy away and telling you to take it, free of charge! Read all three books, or this book, or no books, and implement whatever is helpful to you and your practice. It's my hope that you can apply some of what I've talked about to help get America healthy and redefine dentistry as the key to total health and wellness for everyone.

Life creates either momentum or inertia, which is a synonym for "negative momentum" or moving backward. For years, that negative momentum has pulled dentistry in an adverse direction—negative connotations, negative relationships—but the ground is shifting under our feet.

The movement is already underway; the evidence is everywhere. A recent cover story of *Newsweek* was dedicated to healthy living, and it made frequent allusions to oral health. Dr. Oz lists flossing as one of the top ways to ensure a long life. Flossing!

We're hearing more about dentists and the mouth in the media; it's timely and it's relevant. When the amount of positive messaging in the media is equal to the negativity that's been pervasive for so many years, we'll hit the tipping point.

This morning I was watching the morning news when a new ad came on. "You should watch our news station," it said, "as much as you use *this*." Then they displayed a toothbrush. They were comparing the consumer's daily news intake to a regular dental hygiene routine. Bit by bit, we're coming out of the shadows and entering a totally revitalized, totally redefined era for dentistry.

When something is stretched to an extreme in one direction, it gets catapulted in the other direction fast. I call it the rubber band effect. Dentistry has gotten such a bad rap for so long that once the movement takes legs, it's going to catch fire. Pioneering dentistry is the future. It started with thirty-four pioneers in Cancun. Where it ends remains to be determined.

So how do we reeducate the world about dentistry and what it truly offers? How do we transform the image of the dentist's office from torture chamber to the gateway to total health and wellness? How do we give dentists a makeover, recasting them as the stars of the healthcare movement?

You'll find out how in the next chapter.

Chapter 3 — Takeaways

> ❯ The national movement begins one practice at a time. It starts with you.

> ❯ Most practices operate at 50 percent of their full potential. We've designed a three-year program to turn around that statistic.

> ❯ In Year One, dentists and their teams experience a radical shift in their relationships to money, time, and the people in their lives.

> ❯ In Year Two, dentists and dental team members work on maintaining a Healthy Deserve Level so they can sustain all the success they've achieved.

> ❯ In Year Three, dentists begin looking beyond themselves to pioneer health and wellness worldwide.

> ❯ The journey of a thousand miles begins with a single step. Take the first action today.

> ❯ The movement is already underway. Now's the time to get on board!

CHAPTER 4

DENTISTRY: THE NEW JERSEY OF HEALTHCARE?

'VE LIVED ALL OVER THE UNITED STATES—everywhere from California to New York, and several states in between—but I'm originally from New Jersey. When I tell people I'm a proud Jersey native, I usually get a response along the lines of, "Armpit." That's how Jersey is commonly perceived: the Armpit of America.

In recent years, though, something has changed. Thanks to popular television shows like *The Real Housewives of New Jersey, The Sopranos,* and *Jersey Shore,* people are seeing another side of the Garden State. Like how it's the wealthiest state per capita in the US. And how it isn't all armpit; there's also some pretty lavish living that goes on. Jersey may now be facing other pervasive stereotypes, but it's not "Armpit" anymore. There's been a shift in public perception.

That's exactly what I see for dentistry.

But in order for us to successfully execute that shift, we first have to figure out how and why dentistry is perceived the way it is. How did dentistry get such a bad rap? Why doesn't it get any respect? In this chapter, we're going to discuss why dentistry has commonly been perceived as the Jersey of healthcare, and what to do about it.

It all started back in dental school.

Think back to your days as a dental student. It's probably not a very pleasant memory, right? Of all the dentists I've worked with, not once have I heard anyone laud their time at dental school as "the happiest years of their lives." On the contrary, they talk about their professors tearing them down and telling them all the things they were doing wrong. Dental students are told that they're not going to make it—that they're not good enough. They're bombarded with negative messaging on a daily basis.

There are some schools that are superb institutes of learning where the professors really empower their students, but most professors don't take complex things and simplify them. Instead they take complex things and manage to complicate them further. It's like they're *trying* to make things difficult. When dentists talk about their professors, they don't talk about how much they liked them or how nurturing they were. They talk about how they were unhelpful and discouraging, and how they couldn't wait to get the heck outta dental school. There was not much human connection there, and as a result, there's no love lost when it's time to say goodbye.

You've heard the expression, "Those who can't do, teach." Nowhere is this truer than in dental school. The people in charge are failed dentists who've bought into the notion that the industry is doomed, and they've got the critically low self-esteem to prove it. These are the people training up-and-coming dentists to take the world by storm.

Sure—if that storm is a Category 3 hurricane! I've got several friends who are lawyers, and their personal experience couldn't be more different. They've all got rich memories of law school. They can recall powerful moments shared with their professors, sometimes even down to the details, like specific case names. Not that it was a nonstop joy ride. As the saying goes, "Scared to death, worked to death, bored to death"—that's what happens in your three years of law school. According to my lawyer friends, it's true!

But at the same time, they describe feelings of great respect and admiration for their law school professors. They talk about the kind of expert training they received and what close bonds they forged. Some of them continue to maintain relationships with their old profs, going back to the school for visits and keeping in touch by email. Many have worked alongside their former professors for fundraising and learning initiatives.

In seventeen years of working with dentists, I haven't heard one person say, "My dental professor is my hero. I'm going back to my school to say hi." But I've heard plenty of stories of how it felt to sit in those chairs for years, being constantly degraded and demoted by bitter professors who told them they didn't have what it takes.

People with high self-esteem don't take well to being badgered by people with low self-esteem, but dental students sit there day in and day out, allowing themselves to get beat up psychologically and emotionally. They're caught in the bureaucracy of the system, and so they just sit there and take the abuse. Many dental students are individuals from working class or middle income backgrounds and are the first in their families to attend college, let alone professional or graduate school. So it's possible that they never knew to expect anything more than a negative experience, because they did not have a basis of comparison with other forms of post-graduate education. By contrast, you often see generations of families in medicine, with elitist expectations about experiences, prestige, and income. So medical doctors are more likely to come from wealth and expect to create still more wealth.

Here's the problem: this system sets them up for a legacy of low deserve level in an industry where low self-esteem is the status quo.

So what comes first? Do people with normal self-esteem go into dentistry, only to have their sense of self ravaged by the system? Or does dentistry classically attract people with lower self-esteem, and dental school simply reinforces it? It's hard to say for sure. Either way, dentists come out of dental school a lot worse for wear than when they went in.

In a healthy master-student relationship, there's an expectation that the teacher is going to find fulfillment in training the student. Whether it's a dojo where you learn Taekwondo or the English Department of a top private college, the master is not only gifted in his field; he is also a masterful *teacher*, a nurturer and supporter of the next generation of talent. The dental professor is rejecting the dental student's aspirations and goals, as well as the person he or she is. In so doing, he's not training dentists to close cases. He's training them to get more rejections!

The funny thing—actually, it's not so funny—is that when dental students graduate, their teachers/tormenters essentially shake their hands and say, "Now, you're one of us." Well, this sets up a real problem for the newly hatched dentists—the last thing in the world they want to be is anything like their professors.

There are all kinds of learning that happen in dental school, but unfortunately, primary among them is learning how to be rejected. Sad to say, dentists soak it up like a sponge, and so, after putting in four or more years of sweat, tears, and effort, they're let loose into the real world...and they experience rejection all over again.

When I talk to people who aren't dentists, I try to get them to envision what it's like. "Imagine waking up each day," I say, "knowing that every time you tell someone what you do, they say, 'Gross!' Imagine that reaction, every single time you introduce yourself." When they take a moment to reflect on this, they have a much better understanding of what being a dentist is really like.

We all have some form of low self-esteem. It may be about some aspect of our appearance, or the kind of car we drive, or something we don't think we're good at. For dentists, that self-esteem is tied to the core of what they offer the world. While plenty of people don't like the way their nose looks or the façade of their home, dentists are universally loathed and dreaded, simply for being dentists.

The programming is subconscious, but it can't help but seep in and affect every facet of your life. No wonder dentists have higher suicide rates than other doctors; they live in a world where they're considered to be a dreaded evil! You've been trained as a caregiver—although, according to most of my clients, that training mostly consisted of getting beat up—and once you graduate, you only get *more* beat up. Here you invested over $1 million in your education and setting up a practice, and through it all, you're getting hammered from every direction. People look at you like you're a carrier of some pernicious disease.

Of course, as we both know, you are providing an invaluable service to your patients. But it's an infrequent event when a patient turns to you in the chair and says, "Wow, thank you for making such a difference in the quality of my life!" Ninety percent of dentistry is asymptomatic—there's no tangibility to it—so patients are apt to distrust their dentist. They don't perceive a problem; to them it just seems like the dentist is trying to sell them something they don't need.

It's almost funny how skewed the public perception of dentists can be. First of all, they hear about the one or two quacks who get into the news and give dentistry a bad name—the sole dentist who sexually harasses a patient in the chair or doesn't clean his equipment. Or years ago, the story of a Florida dental office that purportedly spread the HIV virus to patients (the story turned out to be bogus).

The media quickly spins any such story into an industry-wide epidemic, and suddenly, that dentist becomes *all* dentists. To make matters worse, most people assume that their dentist is living next door to LeBron or Kobe in a luxurious gated community. They think dentists make boatloads of cash and enjoy the lifestyle of the rich and famous.

"If only!" most dentists are thinking. It may look that way from the outside, but most dentists can attest that the reality is quite different. From my personal observation, I'd say an estimated 80 percent of dentists are really struggling economically. Twenty percent are living a balanced life, but all the other guys have to sweat it out just to make their payroll. Metaphorically speaking, the common perception is that dentists are married to the New Jersey housewives and vacationing on the Jersey Shore, while in reality they're living in deferred mode and barely scraping by!

The other sad truth is that not only does the public not like dentists; dentists don't like *each other*. Most dentists hate going to programs with other dentists. When we had our "Future of Dentistry" event in Cancun, 99 percent of the attendees made the following confession: "A part of me was dreading coming here, because I don't enjoy hanging out with other dentists, talking about what kind of impression material I use!"

It's sad but true: most dentists don't like being with each other. According to the dentists I work with, when they get together with colleagues in the industry, they always talk about boring stuff that doesn't matter. They have conversations on composite material and other technical aspects of the job. Needless to say, they're usually not the life of the party.

Think of all the ways rejection manifests itself in a dentist's life. They get rejected in dental school, when they're made to feel "less than" and demeaned. They get rejected by their patients and the general public, who think they're molar jockeys and money grubbers. They're even rejected by other dentists, who don't want to be around them. Is it any wonder dentists often live challenged lives? How much rejection can one person take!

Recently, I worked with George, a dentist in Illinois. George wasn't presenting any treatment to his patients. So we went in and helped George set up a healthy mouth baseline. He and his team defined what was healthy and what wasn't, and we went over how he would present it to his patients. He was happy with this improvement, and we sent him on his way to experience far greater growth and success in his practice.

After a few months, I came back to see how George was doing, only to find that he *still* wasn't presenting any treatment. I said, "Why isn't there any treatment coming out of your practice? You've got virtually nothing besides an occasional filling and a crown."

"I guess the jig is up," he said. "When I was on the high school basketball team, I never shot. I was the best shooter in practice, but when it was game time, I never took a single shot. The same is true here. I've got the exact same fear of failure; I'm afraid of being rejected by my patients. All these years later, when I'm chairside, I'm still not taking the shots."

It's easy for a reoccurring event to become the standard by which people operate. It's like a toothache—at the beginning it really hurts, but after a while, you start to get used to it. Rejection works exactly the same way. Because George was afraid of rejection in high school, that same fear followed him around his entire life. It certainly served him well in his profession, which is rife with rejection. Dentists get rejected by the bank for loans, rejected by their team members, rejected by patients. They're battered by the winds of resistance, throughout every day. As a result, they feel sheepish about making even the most basic decision. It is easy to understand why analysis paralysis is the norm for many dentists.

The recurring theme of rejection keeps dentists from doing their job. This just doesn't happen in other industries.

Have you ever heard of an attorney who failed to close a case because the client said, "You know? Actually, I don't think I'll defend the criminal accusation against me after all. Let's just let it go and see what happens." Yeah, right! Even accountants never fail to close cases. They never say, "Let's not file taxes this year and see what happens." Yet dentists are failing to close cases every day, all because quite often they're afraid of facing rejection from their patients.

A lot of dentists know that they're responsible for their inability to produce the results they want to see. That's why I like working with dentists—they're humble enough to see what isn't working. There's an openness there that I haven't seen in other professions.

That's the saving grace of dentistry. That's how we're going to create a shift that will transform the public's perception of dentistry, just like what's happened for New Jersey. Dentists are ready to take a giant leap, precisely because they are *willing to change.*

The first thing that has to change, before we change the public's perception, is the mindset of dentists themselves. The tactical side—what dentists offer—is already there. Dentistry really is fundamental to people's lives, from their aesthetic concerns to overall health and wellness. But before we disseminate this message to the general public, we have to convince the *dentists* that what they're doing is important. We have to reverse a career full of rejection and make them remember who they are: the most important healthcare providers in America!

Here's the good news: because of a career of incessant rejection, dentists are in an ideal position for positive change. The lawyers are going over the side of the boat; law firms are collapsing left and right, and lawyers *still* aren't willing to examine anything. It's simply not in their nature; their careers have depended on them being right. The accountants have no need to change anything, because the tax code is only getting *more* complex; their clients need them more than ever. They're set. And MDs are so used to playing God that they forget they aren't. They don't have the capacity to have the inner dialogue that allows for the possibility of change.

Dentists don't have the arrogance of professions like medicine and law, nor the job security of accountants. It's "death and taxes," not "death and cavities"! You are in a unique position. You've been "beaten into a state of reasonableness," and you're willing to reexamine your life. There's now an opening, a vibrant, viable space for something new. You don't have potential in spite of your history of rejection and bad press; you have potential *because* of it.

Because you've been dragged through experiences of rejection, breaking out of it can be a scary thing. But once you take that first step, magic starts to happen. One of my team members recently told me that she doesn't go for physicals unless her insurance requires it. Instead, she relies on her primary healthcare practitioner, which is her dental internist. She is confident that her hygienist will be able to let her know what's going on in her mouth and, as a result, what's going on in her body. If we can foster this same faith in all of our patients, we will transform perceptions worldwide.

If we keep succumbing to rejection and quietly accept our status, we'll miss out on this defining moment for dentistry. You can stay right where you are, drilling, filling, and billing. What *I'm* saying is that you have access to something far beyond it. And if you get past the rejection and disrespect that's out there, you'll have the opportunity to reverse a lifetime of negative messaging to elevate your profession until it achieves the senior-most position among healthcare practitioners.

It all starts with *you*. You get to choose your future. Not the one that has been given to you by your past. One where you get to say how it goes. You are a practitioner and a caregiver. You are somebody who takes care of not only oral health, but total health. That's the new banner flying over your head, and it's your responsibility to make sure you proudly display that banner everywhere you go.

During our recent event in Cancun, I met a fun couple and told them what I did for a living. Later that day, I ran into them again when I was sitting at a table with the dentists in the conference. The woman called out, "Are those your dentist friends?"

I said, "Yes!"

She crossed her arms and said, "Eww!"

All the dentists just sat there—it was so natural for them to get this response—but I decided not to let it lie. Instead I stood up and went over to my new friends, sat down, and asked the woman why she had responded the way she did.

As it turned out, she really liked her dentist. When she was travelling she had lost a crown, and her dentist had called her back when she needed him. She admitted that "Eww!" was simply a knee-jerk reaction.

By just taking a few minutes, I was able to reeducate this couple about what dentistry really is and why it's important. That's the way to do it—one patient at a time.

Things spread so quickly in today's world with the Internet, Facebook, Twitter, and all the other forms of viral communication. If you do just one communication every day that puts dentistry in a positive light, you've done your job.

It's true that you may feel beaten up from time to time, and you've probably fallen victim to the belief that you're the stepchild of medicine—that you're not worthy of anything more. It becomes a filter through which you process all the input in your life. Now is the time for you to reinvent that filter for yourself. Your inner belief could be, "I'm a respected healthcare practitioner, a dental internist who takes care of people's total health and wellness."

Now when someone questions what you add to their lives, you can gently say, "I know you have that belief and I respect you for it…but may I correct you? I want to share with you what's *really* happening in dentistry and healthcare." Then you can reeducate them, shifting their whole world view.

Rejection has defined your past, but there's no reason it has to define your future. Instead of running away from it, pay attention to it. Reap the benefits of a lifetime of rejection—it's created a humility and receptiveness to change. But don't tune in to rejection any longer. Start tuning in to the future of healthcare instead.

There's a beautiful blank slate of possibility—a new opening carved from the defining moment we find ourselves in. The world has been flattened, and we're allowed to reinvent ourselves. We can now fill the vacuum that exists. People truly don't understand what dentists do or the difference they make, and it's up to us to tell them. We're not in Jersey anymore.

Now is the time. It's time to mold it and shape it...just like a beautiful tooth.

You are the future of dentistry. So you better start paying attention.

If you want to keep up with the way dentistry is going to be revolutionized in the next few years, start looking to the ladies, because they're about to turn the world of dentistry on its head in some awesome ways. As we'll see in the next chapter, it's going to rock your world.

Chapter 4 — Takeaways

> Dental students are bombarded with negative messaging on a daily basis by professors with low self-esteem and a spotty track record of personal success.

> The structure of dental school sets you up for a legacy of low deserve level in an industry where low self-esteem is expected.

> Dentists deal with widespread negativity from the public, who perceive them to be nothing but money-hungry villains wielding painful tools.

> Not only are dentists disliked by their patients, other dentists don't like them, either!

> The longevity of rejection in a dentist's life seems to be never-ending. The *good* news is: this puts you in a perfect position for change! Dentists are, by and large, humble and willing to try something new.

> Take every opportunity to reeducate the public by talking to people about what dentistry really is and where it's headed.

> The future of dentistry is upon us. It all starts with you changing your mindset, and accepting that you're on the way to becoming the most respected healthcare provider in America!

CHAPTER 5

HOW WOMEN ARE TRANSFORMING THE PRACTICE OF DENTISTRY

NOT LONG AGO, dentistry was considered a man's profession. Seventeen years ago, when I first started going to trade shows, I saw the same set of characters in every practice. There was the dentist, almost always a man, surrounded by three to five women—his assistant, hygienist, and office staff. It's like they were all auditioning for the same part: a king surrounded by his ladies in waiting, all carrying tote bags of free goods.

But as we stand on the edge of industry-wide revolution, there's been a dramatic change. In 1920, women in the United States changed the face of American politics when the 19th Amendment guaranteed them the right to vote. Today, nearly a century later, women are about to change yet another fundamental aspect of American life by rising to the forefront of an industry that has traditionally been dominated by men. In this chapter, we'll discuss how women are transforming the practice of dentistry at every level.

It all starts with women dentists.

Dental schools across the US are experiencing a seismic shift in demographic breakdown. Today, 54 percent of students who are graduating from dental school are female. This represents a recent trend over the last decade or so. Between 1995 and 2005, the number of female students enrolling in dental school increased by 32 percent. In 2011, the results are in: it's the first time in history that the majority of dental school graduates are women!

The percentage of practicing dentists is still skewed toward men—82.8 percent of active private practitioners are male, while only 17.2 percent are female. But when it comes to *new* active private practitioners—dentists who have been out of dental school for ten years or less—65.4 percent are male, while 34.6 percent are female. Considering the surge of recent graduates and the rapid retirement of male baby boomers, I expect female dentists to outnumber male dentists by 2017.

What does this mean? It means an exciting new face for dentistry. Women bring something to a dental practice that most men just don't have. They have an inherent caregiver mindset that, sad to say, we guys are often lacking. When people think of a male dentist, they picture him muscling and yanking things. When people think of a female dentist, they think of her gentle touch and nurturing demeanor.

Are these gender stereotypes always accurate? Of course not. There are men who are nurturing caregivers and women who are just as aggressive as their male counterparts. But there are certain unalienable truths, like the fact that women generally have smaller hands, which are less obtrusive in a patient's mouth.

People's perceptions are powerful. There's an abiding misconception that your neighborhood dentist is an old guy peering down at you in the chair with his nose hairs prominently on display. When people think of women, they don't think of nose hairs. So as the public sees more and more practicing female dentists, they're going to be increasingly attracted to going to a dental hygiene appointment.

Dentistry has a lot to offer women today. Many of my female clients work two or three days a week, which allows them to spend time at home with their kids. The profession allows women a lot of flexibility; they can be business owners and professionals and also moms and wives. Not only is it good for them, it's good for the industry, because these women are challenging the status quo of how a practice should be run.

Most male dentists I've worked with live in the "when, then" game. "*When* I have more money, *then* I'll do this." "*When* I have more time, *then* I'll invest more in my marriage." Because many female dentists are also wives and mothers, they have to get things done in a short period of time. They don't want to mess around. As a result, they have crystal-clear, razor-sharp vision.

In my experience, women are often more natural visionaries than men. They come in saying, "This is who I am and this is where I want to go. Now how do I get it done?" They don't analyze and worry things to death. They don't overly concern themselves about failing. They just go for what they want. They're also a lot better at specifics. When I ask men what they want, they either don't know or they muscle up something generic—"More money, more time, less stress." Women will tell me, "I need to work three days a week and make X amount of dollars. I want to have these types of cases, and here's one of the things I need to work on: I'm too friendly with my team. How do I balance this?" They're detail-oriented and clear about what needs to happen, and they're willing to put their butt on the line and declare what they want.

By and large, women don't seem to be as worried about failing as men are, and their identity is less wrapped up in their job. This is a trend I've noticed in and out of dentistry—it may just be a gender thing. But in our industry, it gives women dentists a killer edge.

There's still a glass ceiling, of course. In many parts of the US, dentistry has far to go before it's no longer perceived as an "old boys' network." But as women are becoming increasingly empowered, they're showing up in greater numbers in the dental associations, enhancing their capacity to shape the course of the future. In 1998, the number of women elected as presidents of state dental societies was two out of fifty. In 2006, that number had risen to eight. While there's work to be done before women achieve equal representation, the tides are changing. Female dentists are poised to take the industry by storm.

The irony of the lingering "old boys' network" stigma is that dentistry is not, and never has been, male dominated. Yes, up until recently the majority of dentists have been men, but the industry itself has been powered and empowered by women at every level. Which brings us to the next group of women who are fundamental to a dental practice: the team.

The assistant has the most privileged position of anyone in an office; they have the patient's trust. When the dentist walks out of the room, the patient can—and does—turn to the assistant and say, "Do I really need this? And do I really need it now?" The patient may be suspicious that the dentist is trying to sell them something. The assistant, on the other hand, is their friend.

Then there's the hygienist, who is the only healthcare practitioner who gets to see a patient for two hours in one year. That's huge! People are more willing to go get their teeth cleaned than they are to go get a physical, which places the hygienist in pretty high standing, compared to even medical doctors.

I recently did a focus group where I asked participants, "Why don't you go to your dental office?" They responded, "You know, I *would* go see my hygienist. She's great, and I like getting my teeth cleaned. But I don't want to go in and see some guy who's just going to look into my mouth for two minutes and tell me what's wrong with me."

Even as women are becoming dentists in increasing numbers, the stereotypes can be hard to break. The hidden advantage is that assistants and hygienists—who have traditionally been women—are liked, trusted, and respected by their patients, who feel like they have their best interests in mind.

The support team of any dental practice is populated with relationship-based people, and I don't think I'm the first person to make the observation that women are naturally better at relationships than men. Women are all about creating trust in relationships. If you're a male dentist, having a female team around you can be greatly beneficial.

This goes for your front office administrators, too. Your team leaders and appointment/treatment coordinators *want* to make changes; they just haven't been empowered or been given the direction to do so. As the practice of dentistry is transformed, the front office staff will finally have the power and direction to make big changes and strengthen bonds with every patient who walks in the door.

For years, dental support teams have been squashed by the higher-ups in a practice, but empowering these women is imperative to building strong patient relationships. When they feel respected, they can contribute to the patient in valuable ways. The assistants and hygienists are the ones educating patients, and as the industry is transformed, so is their role. They're not just gum gardeners; they're active participants in educating patients about total health and wellness, and they're living proof that going to the dentist has real value.

Once a support team starts seeing themselves as the dental internists they are, the whole context shifts. They embrace their new identity as dental healthcare providers—the most important providers in the new paradigm of healthcare—and become the catalyst that elevates dentistry in the public sphere.

Then there's the third group of women who play a crucial role in dentistry. These are the spouses—the dentists' wives.

Spouses play a key role in practices. I see a number of baby boomer dentists whose wives do the books, handle the payroll, or manage other parts of the business. Dentistry is one of the few professions where a practitioner's spouse is often involved; I'd say up to 80 percent of male dentists either have a wife who also works in the practice (we see quite a few husband-wife dental teams) or who is actively participating from home.

These women are a great source of support, so empowering them further empowers their husbands, which enables a practice to function at a whole new level. As my ninety-four-year-old grandmother Vera told me years ago, "Find a good woman, Gary. If you trust her, she'll point you in the right direction." The male dentist may be the bus driver, but his wife is his GPS.

As you can see, women are involved at every level of a dental practice, whether they're a dentist themselves or married to one. We're even seeing more women as vendors. Female representatives from Invisalign and Henry Schein are, in many ways, driving this business from the supply side. Thinking of dentistry as a male-dominated profession is an illusion; women are key players at every level.

Unfortunately, they haven't always received the respect they deserve. Either they haven't been empowered as dentists and team members, or their gifts as spouses haven't been honored. But giving women the power and credit they deserve is one of the most potent solutions to reinventing dentistry. They are going to be a primary force in launching dentistry out of the past and into the future, changing how the public perceives it, what it really is, and how it works.

We are entering a new era industry-wide—an era of better, stronger relationships. Women are the obvious candidates to spearhead this shift, since they are innately better at relationships than us men. It's shifting slowly, but we can accelerate it by allowing women to do what they do best: transform relationships, whether it's with the natural trust level they build or with their nurturing, gentle hands. Not only will patients' lives be better, team members' and dentists' lives will be better as well.

You could say that the stars are aligning. Right when dentistry needs a more balanced and holistic world view, women are entering the profession in higher numbers than ever before. The universe is supporting it—there's a convergence between a woman's natural talents and what dentistry needs to pioneer total health and wellness. The entire industry is being catapulted ahead.

To the women I say: this is your revolution. Run with it.

And to the men I say: let them.

Chapter 5 — Takeaways

> The perception of dentistry as a man's profession is an illusion—women are transforming the industry at every level.

> Fifty-four percent of today's dental school graduates are female.

> Women dentists often have a clearer vision of what they want and how they want to achieve it. Then they go after it with less reticence and more energy than their male counterparts.

> The female support team in a practice—the assistants, hygienists, and front office staff—is key to developing relationships with patients and changing the public perception of dentistry.

> A high percentage of dentists' spouses are actively participating in their husbands' practices. Although they've been chronically under-appreciated in the past, their support is crucial to the practices' success.

> Empowering women at a grassroots level will catapult our industry into brand new terrain.

> Women are the harbingers of the dental revolution.

CHAPTER 6

BUT WON'T THIS COST ME MONEY?

A S WE'VE ESTABLISHED, we are in a defining moment for dentistry, or for whichever group of healthcare providers steps up and fills the void that traditional medicine has created. Everything has changed—the economy, healthcare, medicine. Life as we knew it has shifted, and medical doctors are no longer alone at the top of the totem pole. Because the mouth is the gateway to total health and wellness, the most powerful healthcare practitioners in the new paradigm will be the dentists. All they have to do is step up.

But there's a small problem. Many dentists grew up in homes that weren't financially free. They saw dentistry as a way to move up in the world—to achieve the security they'd always dreamed of. For most of them, running a practice has turned out to be a lot harder than they anticipated. They experience a lack of respect on a daily basis; they struggle under the weight of rejection from their patients, team members, and families. While the idea of a dental revolution seems nice in theory, they'd rather stay in their comfort zone of drilling, filling, and billing.

In the last five chapters, we're stirred up all kinds of excitement and possibility for dentists. The future is yours for the taking. And yet, you may be dragging your feet. Maybe you're hesitating, coming up with a million and one reasons why it's not for you. "It all sounds great, Gary," you say. "But I just don't have the money or the time to join a revolution."

It's funny, but as soon as a person has a vision of something better, they often cling to what they have. They're afraid of shaking up their life, even if their life desperately needs shaking up. So they begin operating out of fear. It's always less scary to stay mired in the status quo than to break out into uncharted terrain. But if you don't step out into the future, you'll stay stuck in the past. If you don't challenge yourself to try something new, you're never going to grow.

In this chapter, we're going to surface all those prickly little objections in the back of your mind. It's not just, "How much is this going to cost?", though financial concerns are certainly important. It's all the other quiet grumblings that are holding you back from the life you deserve. "It's just too hard." "I've got bills to pay." "I'm not sure my team will be on board." "My spouse would never go for it." Now is the time to deal with those complaints and debunk them, because they're the only things standing between you and unprecedented success.

Just this morning I was speaking to a new client about what's going on in his practice. "We need to get a handle on our broken and cancelled appointments," he told me. "Can you just give me the quick fix?"

This is how I used to look at dentistry, too. It was all about quick fixes and stop-gap solutions. I used to go into practices and focus on the obvious stuff, like reducing broken appointments and insurance headaches. That was where I stopped looking. It was my whole job. Then, somewhere along the line, I realized I wanted to help my clients make more than a living; I wanted to help them make a life.

Today, after seventeen years of working with dentists, I know that if you want to fix the small issues, you've got to look at the big picture. Now that we're positioning dentistry as the catalyst of a healthcare revolution, it's time to turn our eye to total health and wellness instead of the minutiae of running a practice.

So I asked my client a question. Actually, two questions. "Do you want to continue to put Band-Aids on problems?" I said. "Or do you want to fix them for the long haul?"

He said yes, he'd like the long-term solution.

"Then you've got to embrace the new model of a dental practice," I said. "You've got to move past your old thinking and completely revolutionize your office."

My client voiced some of the usual complaints. He said he didn't have the time or money, and he didn't need any more to do. But here's the thing—there isn't actually more to do. The kind of change we're talking about doesn't take time or money away from something else. Not at all. It shifts your relationships by taking what you're already doing and expanding it. It all starts with expanding what you listen *for*.

Listening *for* is different than listening *to*. Dentists who listen *to* are only paying attention to the words coming out of their patients' mouths. Listening *for* takes it a step further to include what's *not* being said in words—what's underneath the communication. Think of it as *listening 2.0*.

When we work with a dentist and their team, one of the first things we test is what they're listening *for*. There are four levels.

Level 1

This is the lowest level, where 80 percent of practices are. Dentists and dental teams in Level 1 are listening for: "How much money do they have?"

If a patient talks about a luxury cruise he went on, the team assumes he has money. If a patient talks about how her husband lost his job, the team assumes she *doesn't* have money. This results in wallet biopsy dentistry, where the "tissue" being sampled is the person's wallet—dentists essentially test the health of their patient's financial organ before suggesting treatment.

Level 2

The second level of listening is populated by the problem-fixers. These dentists and their teams are listening for: "Are you having any problems?" and "Does anything hurt?" These are the molar jockeys, the ones who are only focusing on what's gone wrong in the mouth and how to fix it. I'd say this encompasses about 95 percent of practices. They can only go as far as problems and pain.

Level 3

Three percent of practices have reached Level 3. These are the dentists, assistants, hygienists, and office staff who are listening for their patients' total wellness. The team is still determining if there are dental problems that need attention, but they're listening from a wider context.

Every time I go to the doctor, I perform a little test by checking the box for "I'm pregnant." And I'll be darned— no one ever asks what trimester I'm in! Dentists who are listening *for* the patient's total physical health are going to notice that checkmark, because they're actually reading the patient's medical history form. They're paying attention to the connections between the mouth and other parts of the body, and they're actively looking at how dentistry intersects with a patient's overall health.

Level 4

The ultimate level is where the pioneers of total health and wellness reside. They've taken it one step further than the dentists in Level 3, because not only are they listening for a patient's total *physical* health, they're listening for their emotional, financial, and spiritual health as well. They're tuned in to the big picture.

One of the practices I work with recently experienced a breakthrough in the fourth level of listening *for*. "Joe," a marine, had been coming in for years, but every time they presented the case for treatment—crowns, fillings, whitening, etc.—he would shrug it off with a firm, "No."

When Joe came to the office for his latest hygiene appointment, there was something different about him. He was smiling, and he looked like he'd lost a few pounds. The hygienist noticed.

"You look great today, Joe!" the hygienist exclaimed. "What's going on with you?"

"I *feel* great," he replied with a grin. "My daughter's getting married in a year and I've been working out. I've already lost twenty pounds!"

Because the hygienist was listening *for* instead of just listening *to*, she understood that Joe wanted to look good for his daughter's wedding. Because she'd spent years building this patient relationship, she knew that this was Joe's only daughter and that seeing her marry a good man—a fellow Marine, no less—was something he'd waited for his whole life.

So she started talking to him about ensuring that his smile looked just as good for the wedding pictures as the rest of his newly trim physique.

Joe's ears perked right up. "What could we do?" he asked.

The hygienist did a shade check, showing him the different shades of white his teeth could be. Then she showed him some of the after shots of other patients who'd had similar work done.

That's all it took to get Joe on board. "Let's do it!" he said. "I want to look the best I possibly can. And I know I'm going to be smiling a lot at the wedding!"

Joe ended up buying eight veneers and having a whole smile makeover. This was the same guy who wasn't ready to buy in the past, but because the hygienist was listening *for* his emotions and his personal motivator (more on that in the next chapter), she was able to provide the exact treatment he needed.

Dentists and dental teams at Level 4 are looking at a patient's *total* picture of health. They're asking them: How's your physical health? Your emotional health? Your financial health? What's going on in your life, and how can we assist?

These questions elicit an ongoing dialogue. When the patient wonders why he's being asked about his total health, the team has the opportunity to explain exactly what's happening in the industry, and how dentistry is being revolutionized. These dialogues work as a catalyst, eventually causing a chain reaction that spreads like wildfire.

These are the four layers of listening *for*. Is a dentist at Level 4 spending any more time with a patient than a dentist at Level 1? No. They're still chairside for the same amount of time, only now, they're asking different questions. Did it cost you more money? Absolutely not! You're doing what you'd be doing anyway; you're simply expanding the vision of what you can see.

Think of it as putting loupes on. When you put loupes on to look into a patient's mouth, it magnifies what you're seeing multiple times. I'm talking about putting loupes on what you are listening *for*. You're spending the exact same amount of time with a patient, but the impact is much more profound. You'll also boost your bottom line.

By changing what you listen *for*, you can't help but make more money. When you pioneer health and wellness, you enhance the perceived value in the patient's mind, so they're going to come back for their hygiene appointments. And when they come to their appointments, they're going to buy treatment because you're actually helping their overall health and wellness; you're not just selling them crowns they don't think they need.

When you listen for something wider, your approach becomes more contextual in nature. This can eliminate the reoccurring issues that you've been trying to deal with in your practice, like cancelled and broken appointments. Listening *for* helps you get to the source of why people don't come to their appointments and why they don't buy treatment when they do show up. In reality, it actually saves you time! Instead of spending every minute chasing down money and trying to patch up the holes in your schedule, your patients are now buying what you offer from the inside out. You no longer have to reel them in and force them to do something; you're providing such an invaluable service that they come to you.

To create this shift, it's important that you move out of poverty thinking and into prosperity thinking. In *Raising Your Healthy Deserve Level*, I talked a lot about this. When we get locked into a poverty mindset, we listen from the place of There's Not Enough. We apply it to everything— not enough money, not enough patients, not enough time. Then we validate our belief system through our filters of There's Not Enough, and, lo and behold, we create Not Enough as a result.

The truth is that there are millions of people in the world, and they all have teeth and gums (if they don't, we can help them with that). Everybody is a candidate for our work. Once dentists have this breakthrough in Year 2 of our work together, they are able to overcome this false objection. They realize that there is more than enough time, money, patients, and teeth for everyone. Instead of putting Band-Aids on symptoms, they've shifted their personal perceptions in relationship to these things, and then they've gotten buy-in from their patients and team members.

What happens next is that the vision expands even further. Once you've gotten your self, your team, and your patients on board, it's time to take the show on the road. Next up: your community, the industry, and the world itself. That last order is a tall one, because the world is recovering from years of negative messaging.

In the past, the media hasn't done dentistry any favors. In the recent movie *The Hangover,* Stu, one of the main characters, is a dentist. When someone is hurt and Stu offers to help, his friends say, "You're not a doctor; you're a dentist." It's that sort of denigration—"Dentists aren't *real* doctors"—that has perpetuated the lack of respect that dentists face on a daily basis. To add insult to injury, I recently heard a radio ad promising that, "Getting a mortgage doesn't have to be as painful as going to the dentist!" Yikes!

But the more I tune in to what the media is saying about dentistry, the more I notice a shift in tone. Slowly but surely, oral health is being recognized as the scientific key to healthy living. I'm seeing evidence on newsstands and online articles. For perhaps the first time in history, dental practitioners are no longer being depicted as ding-dongs; they're beginning to receive the honor and respect they deserve. Dentistry *does* matter. We're bringing it to the forefront and reprogramming the minds of the general public, and it's working.

All these things are happening simultaneously. The media is beginning to subtly change its messaging as the public recognizes the importance of dentistry to overall health. In your practice, you're listening *for*—widening your scope and deepening your context. You're handling problems at their root cause, rather than systematically Band-Aiding each situation.

And yet, some dentists are *still* complaining! They're saying, "This whole 'pioneering total health and wellness' thing is really great, but I'm just too busy."

I give my clients a hard time when they raise the "busy" objection. In my live sessions, I always joke about writing a chapter in my next book called "Why the Back Hates the Front." You know exactly what I'm talking about. In the back, dentists and dental teams are going, "We're *busy* back here! We're handling instruments, cleaning instruments, cleaning and fixing people's teeth. Do you know what they're doing up in the front? They're just sitting around IM-ing their boyfriends. They're Facebooking up there! They're not doing ANYTHING. That's why we hate the front!"

When I go through the whole routine at my events, my clients just lose it. They recognize themselves in the scenario, and they can't help but laugh.

The reason they love it is that they all know they've used the exact same excuse. "We're too busy for pioneering," they claim. "We're just too busy trying to plug all these bleeding points in our patients' mouths." And they're exactly right. They're so preoccupied trying to cover all those bleeding points that they're overlooking the source of why they're bleeding in the first place!

I have some clients who are worried that if they're not handling every single issue that comes up, they'll have nothing to do. "If I wasn't consumed with fixing problems every day," they think, "how the heck would I spend my time?" Our subconscious gets worried that if it didn't have something to complain about, it might get bored. The key is to replace the unproductive actions with productive ones. That means you're not just doing things—you're doing things that matter.

If you're still feeling reticent, you might be struggling with a low deserve level. I have many clients who, after my workshops or seminars, tell me, "Gary, everything you're talking about sounds great. But who am I to deserve to be a pioneer? I'm just your average dentist."

Just like there are four levels of listening, there are five rungs of existence. Deserve level comes in five layers, from lowest to highest.

Layer 1 – "Life is Hard"

The motto of dentists who reside in the lowest layer is: "Life is hard." If anyone tries to make life easy for them, they resist it. Everything is coming through the "Life is hard" filter, and they have a hard time believing there could be another way. Life is a struggle for everybody—that's just the way it is.

Layer 2 – "*My* Life is Hard"

Dentists stuck in Layer 2 have what we call "other people syndrome." They don't believe that *everyone's* life is hard—just theirs. "Other people have great lives," they grumble. "But mine stinks."

Layer 3 – "Life is F.I.N.E."

These dentists are the ones who default to, "I'm fine." They've accepted that their patients are going to hate them, their team is going to be hard to deal with, and the same problems are going to keep cropping up over and over. They're the ones shrugging their shoulders and saying, "You're fine. I'm fine. People are fine." In actuality, they're miserable.

Anytime somebody tells me they're fine, I say, "I'm sorry." For me, F.I.N.E. is an acronym. It stands for Fouled up, Insecure, Neurotic, and Emotional! In that case, why would anyone ever want to be fine?

Layer 4 – "Life is Good"

The fourth layer is one rung above F.I.N.E. These dentists say, "My life is good." They're right—they have a nice life. It's comfortable, and they're reasonably content. But good is the enemy of great. These people are settling for "good" when they could be experiencing far greater fulfillment and purpose.

Layer 5 – "Life is Great!"

This is the top rung, and this is the layer we want to get people to. These are the dentists saying, "Life is great. The world is great. Dentistry is great. And I'm going to do something about it!"

Once you've made it to the fifth layer of a Healthy Deserve Level, you begin to turn your attention outward. In Year 1—the year we covered in *Million Dollar Dentistry*—it's about developing better relationships with your team members, patients, and family. In Year 2, it's about *Raising Your Healthy Deserve Level* and keeping the success you've earned. In Year 3, it's about going beyond yourself and giving back. The paradigm shifts from, "What can I get from this relationship?", to "How can I serve?"

When you reach this level, you begin to appreciate the law of reciprocity. The more you help others get what *they* want, the more you get what *you* want. It's the law of abundance. When you go through these stages and reach this level of mastery in our third year curriculum, life becomes much more fulfilling. It's no longer all about you; it's about the contribution that you make to the world. This actually gives you more peace, joy, and freedom, more money and more time. Basically, all the things you've been desperately groping for now come to you in a natural, effortless flow.

We help our clients get to this point by reverse-engineering. We have them spell out specifically what they want to generate and create, then we work backward. This creates the designed lifestyle versus the deferred lifestyle. There's no "someday when." The someday when is *now*.

This paradigm shift allows dentists and their teams to stop working for their *practice* and make their *business* work for them. It's no longer a job—it's a well-oiled machine. Now that you have more time and more money, you can learn to expand your Healthy Deserve Level, instead of retracting it like a ligament pulling a tooth back to its original position. You can actually *be* with your success. You have created value for your team and patients; you've helped each team member achieve personal, professional, physical, and financial health. Once they get it, it's time to give it away to others. This is the moment when you become a pioneer.

In my first two books, we talked about three stages of the growth process. At first people are uncomfortable being uncomfortable. Then they're comfortable being uncomfortable. Next they're comfortable being comfortable. Now, as we stand on the cusp of a revolution, we've added a fourth stage: uncomfortable being comfortable. These people want to get out there and stir things up. Their attitude is, "What's the next thing for me to do?" They realize that when they get out of their own way and start helping other people, they can make a difference. They're leaving a legacy behind them.

So let's say you're totally on board. You know you're ready to pioneer total health and wellness—to revolutionize not just your practice, but the greater world of dentistry. Great! Now what about your team? How do you let your team know you're serious? That this isn't just the flavor of the month and soon things will be back to normal?

We work closely with our clients to ensure that the changes they make are sustainable for the long term. It's important that each dentist gets agreement from her team once she's created a plan. And it's crucial that you keep your word. When you say you're going to do something, follow through on it. If you don't keep your word, you can restore it by acknowledging you made a mistake: "What I did wasn't aligned with pioneering health and wellness. I apologize. Now let's move on."

If you keep your word, your team will trust you. They'll begin to listen to you with new ears. They'll realize that this *isn't* the flavor of the month. This isn't what you've done in the past; it isn't one of the "ra ra" tricks you may have tried before. This is a commitment you're making as you move forward together into the future. As you're pioneering, you're actively refining, measuring, and monitoring to ensure that every single team member has a role to play.

There are lots of things we do with our clients to keep the commitment and energy level rocking. As a part of our program structure, we designate a "lead pioneer" in each dental practice. This person is responsible for keeping the pioneering spirit alive. The whole team is involved in total health and wellness, but this person is the most engaged in it.

Then we give a flip camera to another team member. We encourage them to use the camera to capture videos of all the successes for health and wellness and post them on YouTube. It might be a clip of the team in action at a trade show. Or it might be a video of an eighty-seven-year-old woman who just got her whole mouth reconstructed; the team asked her what she wanted and gave it to her without putting themselves in the way. Each video is a celebration, and pioneering total health and wellness becomes more real on film.

We also host a contest every year where we award $10,000 to the biggest pioneer. It's a friendly competition; it keeps pioneering fun. We put these structures in place so that total health and wellness becomes a daily, minute-by-minute event. Individual practices perpetuate the trend in different ways. Some put up screensavers on their office computers. Others wear T-shirts that read, "We're pioneers for total health and wellness." The point is for each person to have a key role in keeping it alive.

Pioneering total health and wellness is not for everyone. There are three levels of people in the movement: pioneers, frontier people, and settlers. The pioneers are leading the pack, clearing the brush away. They want to take action and revolutionize the industry. The frontier people come right behind them to lay down the road. They perpetuate what the pioneers have begun. The settlers come last; they put up houses and libraries and schools, settling the land once it's habitable. You may consider yourself more of a settler than a pioneer. That's okay. We'll meet you wherever you are.

Whether you work with us directly or not, the principles in this book are yours to apply however you see fit. Dentists and dental teams across the country have taken the lessons they learned from my first two books and produced huge results in their practices. Now you can do the same. I'm not going to chase you down the street and demand that you become a pioneer for total health and wellness, but by laying it out in this book, the vision becomes clearer—a vision you can step into.

Now that we've overcome your objections, it's time to get your patients on board. In the next chapter, we'll get into the head of your patients and figure out what motivates them. Because it's not about change; it's about transformation.

Chapter 6 — Takeaways

> If you want to fix the small issues in a dental practice, you've got to look at the big picture.

> Expanding what you listen *for* will revolutionize the way you work with your team and your patients.

> Once you've made it to Level 4 of listening *for*, it's like putting loupes on. You're spending the same amount of time as you did before, but your results are magnified many times over.

> Move from poverty thinking to prosperity thinking. Don't let your belief system be shaped by "There's not enough." There *is* enough—time, money, patients, and teeth.

> Deserve level comes in five layers. Once you've reached the fifth level, you begin to want to give back to your community, industry, and world.

> Getting your team on board is about making sure that everyone has a key role to play. We also put structures in place—flip cameras, T-shirts, screensavers, a $10,000 contest—to keep the spirit of pioneering alive.

> Whether you define yourself as a pioneer, frontier person, or settler, there's room in the movement for you. So step right up and take your place!

CHAPTER 7

GETTING THE PATIENTS ON BOARD

A S THE DENTAL REVOLUTION transforms our profession, getting buy-in from the public is essential. The catalyst for the movement takes place in each individual practice, in the relationship between the people performing the work and the people having the work done. It all starts with those ever-elusive and often frustrating characters you can't live without: your patients.

The Ancient Greek physician Alexander of Tralles once said that a doctor "should look upon the patient as a besieged city and try to rescue him with every means that art and science place at his command." That's exactly what you have to do—rescue your patient from a lifetime of inaccurate and misguided information about what dentistry really is, and what it means for them.

In this chapter, we're going to talk about how to get your patients on board. What motivates patients to go to their dentists and pay for treatment? Perhaps more importantly, what causes them *not* to go?

It's the responsibility of the dentist and dental team to educate the patient—and in many cases, to reeducate the patient—about dentistry. For years, our industry has plodded along in a linear—though not necessarily logical—progression. It goes like so: The dentist looks in a patient's mouth. He understands what the problem is. The patient doesn't. He tries to tell the patient to pay a lot of money for a painful treatment of a problem the patient doesn't even perceive. The patient balks and walks. End of scene.

Old school dentistry was founded on the assumption that patients remain in the dark; they don't understand the problem and they don't understand the solution, all for one simple reason: no one has taken the time to explain it to them. And who in their right mind wants to sit in a chair while being bombarded with a laundry list of expensive treatments when they don't even know why they need them?

Over the last ten years, I've interviewed thousands of patients. What I learned surprised me. Patients don't tell the truth about why they're not saying "Yes" to dental treatment. I once did a focus group with thirteen men and women where I asked, "Why don't you go to your hygiene appointments?"

A woman raised her hand. "I'll tell you why," she said. "I wake up in the morning and see that I have a dental appointment. I don't even shower. I just throw my clothes on and go. Then I walk into my dentist's office, and a woman starts asking me question after question. 'Are you having any problems? Is anything hurting? Did you floss?' Of course I didn't floss. I didn't even shower!

"Then my dentist comes in, who I'm pretty sure doesn't even know my name, and starts telling me what's wrong with me. And I didn't even think there *was* anything wrong with me; I thought I had a great smile. So it's going to cost me a thousand bucks to fix issues I didn't even know were issues. To top it all off, they're running late, which is going to take time out of my day. It's a beautiful morning—one of the last warm days before a long winter—and I'm spending it staring at my dentist's ceiling. Now you tell me: why the heck would I do that?"

I said, "Good point!"

In that moment, I had a huge realization. When's the last time you bought something you didn't think you needed that a) costs thousands of dollars, b) takes time out of your day, and c) will probably hurt? The woman in my focus group was exactly right! Why the heck *would* you do that?

The public perception of dentists is that all we do is tell people what's wrong with them—we don't really provide value. *We* may understand that they have a problem, but people only buy solutions to problems that *they* know they have. If, on the other hand, we tie the dental solution to what they value in life, then we can change the equation.

Strictly speaking, there are three things that dentistry provides: health, function, and aesthetics. But these are still means to an end. Think of it like buying a drill. You don't buy a drill for the drill itself; you buy it to make holes. Actually, you don't even buy it to make holes. You buy it because you want to use it to build something bigger.

Health, function, and aesthetics are the drills that provide something else. Health provides longevity and well-being. Function provides pain-free living—being able to eat, chew, sing, talk, and kiss with no problems. Aesthetics provides an opportunity for, in the words of Justin Timberlake, "bringing sexy back." A beautiful smile boosts your confidence and improves your relationships.

As dentists, it's up to us to provide value to our patients. How we provide that value is of the utmost importance. This is where the paradigm shift comes in. What we're doing is creating a tsunami-sized vacuum where, instead of having to push dentistry *on* our patients, the patients are actually *pulling dentistry toward them.* To explain this shift, I want to begin by talking about…root planing and scalings.

Not the sexiest part of being a dentist, right? As we all know, root planing and scaling is the treatment for someone who's experiencing pocketing. But the minute you say "pocketing" to a patient, they tune out. The term means nothing to them—they don't care. However, if you are able to couch it in terms they understand, you'll have a lot more success.

Begin by giving your patient a clear definition of the problem. Instead of saying, "You've got pocketing," say, "You have gum recession. What that means is that you have bacteria below your gums that are eating away at your bone. If we don't step in to intervene, you could lose your teeth." By spelling out the consequences, you've painted a clear picture for your patient of the potential cost of inaction.

Then, present your patient with the solution. Don't say "root planing and scaling"—that's empty jargon to their ears. Instead, try, "We're going to gently clean below the gum line so that we stabilize the bacteria and eliminate the bone loss, so you can keep your teeth for a lifetime."

You've now presented the solution in crystal-clear terms, and you've also explained why this treatment is necessary if they want to keep their teeth.

That's the big picture. Think of it as a blueprint for engaging the patient on a deep level so that they *want* to buy what you're offering, versus pushing treatment on people only to have them decline it.

Now let's break it down. I've further simplified the process into five easy steps. If you and your team follow these steps, it will dramatically alter the way your patients experience dentistry.

STEP 1 – Establish a Healthy Mouth Baseline

In the old model, the patient's perception was that their dentist was just going to try and sell them commodities—crowns, fillings, cleanings, and the like. But when dentists establish a healthy mouth baseline in their office, it completely shifts the paradigm. Now the patient understands that the whole dental team is going to let them know what is and isn't healthy from a factual standpoint.

In the old days, a patient listened through automatic filters. Everything her dentist or hygienist said came through sounding fuzzy, because she didn't understand what they were really providing. When you establish a healthy mouth baseline—and not just establish it, but print it, laminate it, and put it up in your treatment room and reception area—you're telling your patient exactly what dental health entails: freedom from disease, decay, infection, crowding, and anything else you and your team decide to include.

This is where it all begins. Now the patient sees that

you're coming from a place of total health and wellness, and that dentistry isn't reactive; it's proactive. They're ready to listen to what you have to say. Now your patient doesn't feel the pain of you telling them what is *wrong with them*; they decide for themselves. Way better!

STEP 2 – Listen for the Patient's Personal Motivator

Dentists often make the mistake of selling a patient what *they* want to sell them, but if you can determine what the patient is motivated by, then they'll buy treatment from you. This is Step 2 of the process.

To help the dentists we work with shift their patients' perceptions of dentistry, I created a simple, radical common sense tool called "locating the personal motivator." In essence: you have to understand what motivates your patient.

Everybody is motivated by something different. That's why you have to adopt a unique approach with each patient. Remember Joe the marine from the previous chapter? The hygienist was able to locate his personal motivator—looking good for his daughter's wedding—by listening *for*.

Take another example. Let's say I'm your patient. Because you've done a good job of listening *for* over the years, you know that my personal motivator is longevity and health. I'm forty-six years old; I no longer feel immortal. I see the deterioration of seventy-year-old family members, and I realize that I've only got twenty-four more years of decent health. I've also got a six-year-old son and a delectable wife, and I want to be around for him and her for the long run. All of those factors motivate me to take good care of myself.

Because you care about my total health and wellness, you know that I had pancreatitis a few years back and that it was hell on earth. You also know that 62 percent of people who have soft tissue inflammation have a higher susceptibility to pancreatic cancer. Wouldn't you know it—despite writing three books on dentists and dentistry, when I come in for my biannual checkup, my gums are inflamed.

If, during my hygiene visit, you tell me that my oral condition substantially increases my chance of more pancreatic distress and negatively affects my long-term health, do you think I'm going to pay attention?

You bet!

If you present the statistic that I am 62 percent more susceptible to pancreatic cancer because of inflammation in my mouth, am I going to take action? No doubt about it.

Now, if you say to me, "You have five-millimeter pockets and seventeen bleeding points, and you need root planing and scaling for $1,500," I won't be nearly as receptive. But if you frame it in terms of my personal motivator—maintaining my health—I'm going to listen. If you show me that dentistry is going to help me live a longer life, I'll do whatever it takes. In fact, I just did. I invested several thousand dollars in dental treatment because I want to be around for my son and wife for as long as possible. For me, that's worth any amount of money.

It's important to listen for personal motivators with each individual patient, every time they come in. To go back to

Joe's story: if the hygienist had assumed that nothing had changed since his last visit—that looking good just wasn't a personal motivator in his life—she would have missed a golden opportunity. Instead, she began that visit fresh and listened anew for what his personal motivator might be. As it so happened, his personal motivator *had* changed, and she was able to give Joe exactly what he wanted: a beautiful new smile so he could look his best on his daughter's (and his) big day.

STEP 3 – Apply the PCS™ Method

Ninety percent of dentistry is asymptomatic. That means nine out of ten patients who need treatment have no way of knowing they need it. Their teeth don't look bad, their mouth doesn't hurt, and there are no symptoms associated with their problems. Studies have proven that people don't buy solutions to problems they don't think they have.

That's why it's important that you educate your patient by highlighting the problem. In Step 3, you're ready to build your case because now you can tie the problem back to the personal motivator you located in Step 2. That's when you launch the PCS™ method: Problem, Consequence, Solution.

First, the problem. Let's say the patient has disease, decay, and infection, which was determined by the healthy mouth baseline you set. So you've identified what's wrong in the patient's mouth.

Problem is, most dentists and dental teams don't want to be the bearer of bad news. So they minimize the problem. "Well, you have a little infection here," they say, "and maybe some disease. And there's a tiny crack in that tooth—but just a small one." By minimizing the problem, they minimize the patient's motivation to take action. The patient thinks, "So what? I'll just go home and put some peroxide on it."

Can you imagine someone having that kind of response if their MD told them they had cancer? Of course not!

It's vital that the patient understand the cost of inaction. That's when you move into the C of PCS: consequences. Don't lighten or soften it; you owe your patient the whole truth and nothing less. Tell them, "You've got disease, decay, and infection, and if it goes untreated, it's only going to get worse. Not only on an oral health level, but on a total health level." Tie it back to the patient's personal motivator.

Then, instead of going right into the solution, say, "Do you have any questions?"

Your patient usually has one of two questions, and sometimes both: "How do I get the decay and infection out of my mouth?" and "How much is it going to cost me?" By giving them the chance to ask you those questions, you've shifted the energy in the room. No longer are you *selling* dentistry; rather, people are raising their hands, coming to you and saying, "How do I fix this problem? What do I have to do?", which gives you the perfect opportunity to say, "Glad you asked. Let me share that with you."

Now it's time for the S of PCS: solution. This is the moment when you explain, by thoughtful and attentive patient education, how the solution is not going to be more painful than the problem. If the patient thinks that they've got minimal disease and decay, and you propose a root planing and scaling at $1,500, they may be thinking that the solution sounds way bigger than the problem!

This is where the assistant has a crucial role to play. When the dentist leaves the room, the patient will often turn to them and say, "Do I need to get this done now?" We teach our assistants *not* to say, "Yes, you should get it done now." That ends up sounding pushy. Instead, we teach them to say, "It would be irresponsible of me to say, 'No, you don't.'" Then the onus is on the patient to make the responsible choice.

I often remind my clients to have compassion for their patients. Going to the dentist can be very stressful. Dentists are desensitized to it because they see dozens of patients every day, but being in a dental chair can be incredibly intimidating. I've had patients tell me it's worse than getting pulled over by a cop! You're lying prostrate in the chair, vulnerable, with your mouth open wide—you might as well be naked—while the dentist looms over you, large and dominating. The only thing that's missing is a strap to hold you down in the chair, straitjacket style!

Meanwhile, the patient is filtering everything through the lens of, "How much is this going to cost?" They're banking on the fact that the dentist is making a lavish living off their crowns and fillings. One dentist told me that when he told a patient to open wide, she responded, "You're going to find your next Porsche in here!"

It's up to you and your team to make your patient understand that you're not trying to buy a sports car or renovate your family home; you're trying to provide what *they* want and need. Not everyone processes things the same way, so you've got to tailor your approach to the individual patient.

They have to see, hear, and feel it. Are they visual, auditory, or tactile? Do you need to paint the picture of total health and wellness in words or images? The tools you use—like intraoral cameras for visually oriented patients—will be important. And no matter who the patient is, they need to hear it verbally five times. That brings us to Step 4.

STEP 4 – Fire Up the Five-Time Trust Transfer

At my live events, I talk about how to get treatment from the back to the front. It's one of the biggest problems dental teams face. I've had dentists say to me, "Well, we closed it in the back, but by the time the patient got to the front, those darned front desk people—they blew it!" Meanwhile, the patient never bought it in the back in the first place.

That's where the five-time trust transfer comes into play. The patient has to hear the problem, consequence, and solution (PCS), tied to the personal motivator, five times.

Here's how the five-time trust transfer works:

1st – The hygienist or assistant speaks it to the patient.

2nd – The hygienist or assistant speaks it to the doctor in front of the patient.

3rd – The doctor speaks it to the patient.

4th – The hygienist or assistant speaks it to the treatment coordinator in front of the patient.

And finally,

5th – The treatment coordinator speaks it to the patient.

What's brilliant about the five-time trust transfer is that the two most trusted people are now originating the treatment. The assistant is the number one trusted person in a dental office, and the hygienist is number two—and the most influential in the patient's mind. The patient feels like these two people, who are more often than not women, are "on their side."

This is one of the keys to transforming public perception at lightning speed. We're putting the revolution in the hands of the people who elicit no suspicion in the minds of the patient. No one suspects the hygienist of trying to sell more crowns so she can buy her next Porsche!

STEP 5 – Fitting the Treatment into the Patient's Lifestyle

Now that the patient understands what dentistry is and how the roles of the dentist, hygienist, assistant, and team members are going to play out in her total health and wellness, the only step that remains is working together to co-create a treatment plan that is a perfect fit for her lifestyle.

When you go in to buy a car, they don't ask you how much you want to pay for the total car. They ask, "How much do you want to spend per month?" No wonder patients go running for the hills when we hit them with a lump sum of $5,000! But for some reason, most dentists still haven't learned this lesson.

Even after we get patients to buy into their treatment and see the value of it, only 20 percent like to pay the full amount with a discount. The other 80 percent want to break it down into more manageable payments. That's why every practice should have a dedicated person who deals with the money and breaks treatments down per month. This person should *not* be in the back—issues of money should always be reserved for the front.

We typically encourage our clients to use third-party financing. Most dentists don't. They say to the patient, "Do you want a credit card?" What we do is break it down per month and make the dentist look like the hero by saying, "By using Care Credit, you get twenty-four months interest-free, and that $5,000 case is $199 a month with no money down."

To which the client inevitably replies, "$199? I can get rid of disease and decay and get my teeth straightened and whitened for less than two hundred bucks a month? Sign me up!"

And the rest is dental history.

I've seen this simple five-step process transform hundreds of dental practices across the country. At the heart of this shift is your new and improved relationship with your patients. We're not talking about change; we're talking about transformation. By following these five steps, you've shifted the paradigm and completely transformed the way your patients think of dentistry, and the way they respond to you.

The process I just outlined is how to engage your *existing* patients. But what about new patients? How do you engage them in the new model?

In one sense, your new patients are a blank slate—you get a fresh, clean start when it comes to reeducating them about dentistry. But keep in mind that new patients came from somewhere else, and their preconceptions (and misconceptions) of dentistry might be stronger than any of your current patients', and possibly a lot more negative. It's up to you to retrain them. The way to bring their expectations and education up to speed is through a three-step process: VIP intake form, VIP interview (where you interview each other and set expectations), and a trust exam.

By implementing these three tools, you'll have a process that allows you to integrate new patients into your family of patients, rather than having them run amuck and bog the system down. They'll understand that your office is different from others they may have been to. You're offering a package experience—you're not cutting teeth and putting in porcelains; you're not gum gardeners or molar jockeys. Instead, you're offering health and wellness for everyone who walks through your doors. Once they know that, they'll be glad they did!

What we've essentially done is reinvent the flow that happens inside of a practice. If you don't break out of the old model, you'll keep bumping into the same problems of low case successes and low patient retention. The flow in the new model helps you grow your practice versus continuing to invest time and energy in the things that don't work.

In the new model, the patient no longer feels like they're getting pulled over by a cop when they're in the dental chair. They're not being dominated; they're being contributed to. Whereas they used to feel like they were getting taken advantage of, now they think of the dentist's office as a place where they get loved and cared for—where their total health and wellness is a top priority.

Now that you know how to engage your patients, let's talk about how to get your team members on board. When it comes to transforming dentistry worldwide, it doesn't take a village—it takes a team, as you'll discover in our next chapter.

Chapter 7 — Takeaways

> For most patients, going to the dentist means taking valuable time out of their day to be told what's wrong with them and how much fixing it is going to cost. No wonder they skip appointments!

> Engaging your patients means reeducating them about how and why dentistry provides value by using a five-step process.

> First, establish a healthy mouth baseline. Make sure every team member and patient in your practice knows exactly what a healthy mouth looks like, and what an unhealthy mouth looks like.

> Second, listen for the patient's personal motivator. Find out what they want and need, and show them how you can provide it.

> Third, apply the PCS™ method. Show them the problem, consequences, and solution, and speak in a language they understand.

> Fourth, utilize the five-time trust transfer. Make sure the patient hears their need and the proposed treatment for it five times.

> Fifth, fit the treatment into their lifestyle. Make it easy for them to get a healthy mouth and a beautiful smile.

> When you take on new patients, be sure to include an intake form, interview, and trust exam.

> The time is now to become responsible for a new level of accountability in health and wellness. Make sure your patients know that transformation is on the way, and that it starts in your office!

CHAPTER 8

YOUR PATIENTS TRUST YOUR TEAM MORE THAN YOU!

E'VE SURFACED YOUR OWN OBJECTIONS to joining the dental revolution—and dissolved them. We've discussed what motivates your patients and how to ensure that they're on board. Now let's talk about the people who have the power to make or break your newly formed vision: your team.

Your team members are the key players in industry-wide transformation. They're the be-all and the end-all of reprogramming dentistry. Why?

Because your patients trust them more than they trust you!

That's right. You spent years slaving away in dental school, learning everything there is to know about teeth and gums, and you've got the DDS after your name to prove it. But guess what? No matter what you say to a patient, when you talk, they're listening through a filter.

A filter is an automatic and subconscious belief in a person's mind. Whatever you say, they're going to process it to make their belief right. That's how filters work; they make outside data match up with an internal belief system so that there are no discrepancies.

Even if a dentist has the best of intentions, most patients are still mired in the mindset that he or she is making a killing off every crown and filling. Like the woman from the last chapter, they're convinced that dentists are looking for their next Porsche in a patient's mouth. I don't care how trustworthy, kind, and caring you are, that's still the background conversation going on in the minds of most of your patients. There's an enduring misperception that dentistry is being done for the *dentist's* benefit, not the patient's.

If we want the ongoing dental revolution to continue its course, it's vital that we get the patient to understand the words coming out of our mouths. In fact we've developed a simple quota system to ensure we're on the right track. We've found that when most dentists talk to their patients, the patient is only truly hearing one word out of ten. If ten words come out of your mouth and the patient only connects to one, we're never going to get anywhere!

But when you expand your perspective to include other team members, the equation changes. If ten words come out of an assistant's mouth, the patient believes all ten. If ten words come out of a hygienist's mouth, they believe nine. And if ten words come out of a front office administrator's mouth, they believe seven.

Once you do the math, you'll see why it just doesn't make sense to continue to spend time having the dentist do all the work!

There are two models of dental teams: the old and the new. In the old model, team members felt devalued and unimportant, stuck in a dead-end job. They went through the motions every day, but really they felt like puppets with the dentist pulling all the strings.

When I worked with practices in England, I shared with dentists how the hygienist should be the one to originate the PCS™ method and educate the patient on total health and wellness. Every dentist replied, "Absolutely not. No way that's happening here." It was a breakthrough moment for me, because I realized how deeply ingrained the hierarchy has become in Western culture. If you're a doctor, you don't delegate much, if at all. That's just the way it is.

But the old model isn't working. It hasn't been for some time. What we're talking about in this book is a dramatic pivotal shift in how the general public perceives dentistry, and the only way to make that shift is to bring dental team members to the forefront. In the battle to transform dentistry, your team is on the front lines.

The new model is vibrant with potential and opportunity. It's going to revitalize your team and give each individual an important role to play in pioneering total health and wellness.

Many practices are trying to put in systems and processes that change their patients' beliefs or eliminate their filters, which is time-consuming and ultimately ineffective. Our approach is: why not take the people they trust, whose influence they already accept, and build systems around those people instead? You'll make a bigger, faster impact, and you'll get off the treadmill of trying to forge through the filters that people have been living with for a lifetime.

If you can shift to the new model, where patients listen to ten out of ten words instead of one out of ten, you'll be working smarter, not harder. Your case acceptance will skyrocket, and your life will become easier as a result. Your patients understand the true impact of dentistry because they are now beneficiaries of genuine patient care. The old adage is true: people don't care how much you know; they want to know how much you care. They'll get that from a team member before they get it from a dentist.

In this chapter, I'm going to lay out the roles of every team member according to the new model—their vital purpose and how they can best fulfill it. Let's start with the dental assistant.

The assistant is the most trusted person in a dental office, and in the old model, the least utilized. Up until the dental revolution, many assistants weren't thrilled with what they were doing—it was a good job, but not great. They didn't see any opportunity for growth, and they often doubted their own abilities. For years, we'd walk into a practice and hear them say, "I'm just an assistant." It was so prevalent that we actually created a new term: "NJAs," for Not Just Assistants!

A dental assistant does so much more than hand instruments to the dentist and turn rooms. There's actually *huge* opportunity for growth. It's all about trust. The patient trusts the dental assistant more than anyone else in the office—more than the front desk people, more than the hygienist, and more than you, the dentist.

As we observed hundreds of dental practices, we noticed something interesting. After the doctor presented a case, she would walk out of the room to go prepare for the next patient as the assistant finished up. Nine times out of ten, the patient would then turn to the assistant and ask one of three questions: "Do I really need this?", "Do I really need this *now*?", and "Is she a good dentist?" This put the assistant in a prime position for guiding the patient toward right action.

Unfortunately, the assistant had been invalidated in front of a patient or treated as "less than" by the dentist. So when the patient asked these questions, they would respond with uncertainty and hesitation. The buying decision was made by the patient in that moment, and they decided not to buy treatment. You can have the greatest treatment coordinator in the world, but the patient is going to trust the assistant before they trust anyone in a sales position.

In my work with practices, I've taken this naturally existing trust relationship and expanded it, using it as a platform to elevate the assistant's position. They're not just dental assistants any longer—they're the doorway to dentistry's transformation. It all begins by widening their personal perspective.

Remember what TVs were like ten or even five years ago? They were small and the screens were narrow. Compare that to the beautiful widescreen TVs people have today, with Blu-ray high definition and 3D imaging. Is there a difference? You bet!

It's time that dental assistants see the big picture. We want to widen their view and give them greater clarity about the impact they have in a practice. In the old model, their scope was 2D—they felt like all they did was hand instruments to the dentist and turn rooms. But in the new model, they've got 3D responsibilities: Developing Dentistry through Discernment!

The fundamental building block of discernment is good education. We share with every dental assistant we work with: "You are the most influential educator in a dental office. If you unleash that influence with every patient every day, and we can get other dental assistants in other offices to do the same, it's going to jumpstart the revolution."

Think of your assistant as your co-pilot and partner. That doesn't mean she's better than you; it simply means she's got more of an influential role with the patient. Your job is to empower her. I'm not saying that assistants should diagnose patients or replace the dentist in any way. What I'm saying is that empowering dental assistants on a grassroots level will allow them to educate the patient with confidence and certainty, leading to higher levels of patient trust and case acceptance.

One thing I really appreciated about practices in England is that they refer to dental assistants as "dental nurses." I think we should adopt the same term in the States. Nurses are highly trusted—probably more trusted than doctors these days. If dental assistants thought of themselves as dental nurses, I guarantee they'd feel a lot more confident in the power they have.

Our goal is to empower assistants so that they don't have a reactive role to the doctor, but a highly proactive one. As the number one patient influencer, they are able to utilize that inherent strength to not only improve the practice and the patient's life, but to shift how patients relate to dentistry and dentists in general.

Next up in the dental team lineup is the hygienist, the second most trusted person in a dental office. It's not uncommon to hear, "I love my hygienist, but I hate my dentist. When I go in for a cleaning, I try to get away with just seeing my hygienist and avoiding the doc!" And yet, despite the friendly relationships they enjoy with their hygienists, many patients only see them as "cleaning girls" or "cleaning guys."

When we work with hygiene departments, our goal is to widen their perspective, just like we do with dental assistants. We educate them out of narrow, limited thinking and widen their scopes so that they see how crucial they are to pioneering total health and wellness. We want our hygienists to view their role in 3D: Developing Dentistry through Detection.

The hygienist is the first person to detect what's going on in a patient's mouth. In the old model, hygiene teams only tended to the soft tissue. As a part of our methodology, we ask hygienists to devote a third of their one-hour hygiene visit to educating patients on hard tissue health as well. Because the hygienist is trusted, when they originate the problem and consequences of a patient's hard tissue health, the patient listens. Then the dentist gives the solution, and the hygienist affirms it.

Now we're getting into the oral systemic connection. Hygienists are the harbingers of Developing Dentistry through Detection because they're the ones educating the patient on the mouth as the gateway to total health. Take, for example, the cutting-edge technology where you can swab saliva and tell a lot about diabetes, cancer, and other diseases. If the hygienist is the person taking that swab, they've suddenly got crucial information that the patient wants and needs.

The role of the hygienist is even more important in light of the current changes in healthcare. The Obama administration plans to cut costs of $200 billion a year from healthcare over the next ten years. One of the places they're going to trim expenses is in the administrative costs. The way things stand today, you might go to six different doctors for six different complaints, and every time they'll have to start from scratch compiling your medical history. That's why our nation is transitioning to a system where every patient has a centralized medical record—the hope is that it will save millions of dollars in administrative costs, not to mention save time and avoid errors and duplication of efforts.

In the new healthcare paradigm, in a world where dentists have positioned themselves as the primary healthcare provider, the hygienist is more powerful than ever before. They now hold the key to detecting sickness and disease in its early stages. Patients understand that a visit to the dental office no longer means simply a cleaning; it means their total health is going to get checked out. And because they're listening *for*, hygienists really understand the emotional aspects of their patients and how this ties into holistic wellness in mind, body, and soul.

When we work with hygiene teams, we help them understand that the words coming out of their mouths are incredibly important. According to our research, the patient is listening to nine out of ten of those words, and sometimes nine point five. So instead of talking about the latest reality TV show or what's new around town, why not proactively share a picture of total health and wellness?

Keep in mind that the hygienist is probably the only medical practitioner who actually spends two full hours with a patient each year, affording ample opportunity for patient education. In today's fragmented healthcare system where people sometimes wait hours for a fifteen-minute checkup, I can't think of many doctors who can say that!

When we get hygienists out from under the "cleaning lady" moniker and empower them to think like dental internists, magic happens. Suddenly, there's added value to going to the dentist's office. The patients love it because now they can kill two birds with one stone—they're going to get their teeth cleaned, but they know that their hygienist is also going to check up on their total health and wellness. They didn't even have to schedule a physical and go sit in a waiting room for half a day!

The hygienist's new role as dental internist is pivotal in helping the dental revolution take off. In the new model, dentists effortlessly glide into a more senior position in the healthcare paradigm, because it just makes the most sense. Patients don't have to seek out a naturopath—which can be daunting, considering there aren't many and they're sometimes a good distance away—and they don't have to go to a chiropractor, which many people still feel dubious about. All they have to do is go to their trusted dentist's office, which they were going to do anyway. If there's any issue with their health, it will be identified. The hygienist is the first stop on the path to prevention.

The hygiene department is the pinnacle of total health and wellness as we move forward into the future. Hygienists have an inherent desire to get people healthy and well, and to make sure their patients look and feel good. By tapping into this innate goal, you're enabling them to do exactly what they want to do. You're essentially giving them the tools they need to do the job they love.

The next team members are the front office administrators—the appointment coordinators and treatment coordinators. In the old model, the patient listened to seven out of ten words that came out of their mouths. We've been able to bring them up to almost nine point five out of ten through some simple paradigm shifts.

Let's begin with the appointment coordinator. This is the patient's first point of contact with the office. As such, it's an important position. Yet the average dental practice is severely understaffed in this area. They usually have one person when they need two, or two when they need three.

It's one of the most common problems we encounter in dental practices—one person is trying to do too many things. Most often, it's the appointment coordinator who is forced to also wear the treatment coordinator hat. She can't focus on coordinating appointments because she's juggling too many things at once. As we've learned, it is absolutely imperative that there be at least one dedicated appointment coordinator in every office.

Why is such a critical need so frequently overlooked? Because most dentists are living in the "when, then" mindset: "*When* I make more money, *then* I'll add more people." What they don't realize is that in their attempt to keep their payroll low, they're missing out on world-class customer service…and a lot more profit.

When you look at the average annual value of a patient in a dental practice, it can be anywhere from $1,000 to $1,500. So for every hygiene appointment that a patient misses, the practice is losing $500 to $750. That's a lot of money! That's why it's essential that you have a stellar appointment coordinator in place to process new patients, as well as existing patients, through recare and case acceptance. If you look at your payroll as return on investment, you'll see why appointing one or more people exclusively to the role of appointment coordinator is more than worth it—even if it means adding an extra salary to your payroll.

From the dentist's perspective, it's a payroll issue. But there's another issue that can come into play, this one from the team's perspective. Let's say you have a fantastic appointment coordinator in place, but your practice is growing and you really need to hire a second person to assist with the increased patient flow. What sometimes happen is that a security issue arises—the other team members feel threatened by the new person. Before, they felt necessary to the work of the practice; now they feel replaceable. This dynamic can explain the "revolving door" of hiring that plagues many practices. When dentists tell me, "We can't find good people," it's often because the other team members didn't subconsciously welcome the new person.

But if the appointment coordinator is made to feel valued and important, it eliminates the problem. It all starts by empowering them to do their job in 3D: Developing Dentistry through Demeanor.

As the first person the patient interacts with on the phone or in person, the appointment coordinator sets the tone for the entire visit. If they are positive and welcoming, the patient will feel relaxed and comfortable. If they are curt and harried, the patient will respond in kind.

Most of the time, when we call dental offices to follow up after a live event, it's obvious that we're an intrusion on their day. The appointment coordinator doesn't know who we are or why we're calling, and they usually put us on interminable hold. I've got nothing against these individuals—they're doing their job the best way they know how. But when they're having to juggle fifteen different things at once, no wonder they can't give a high level of personal attention to each patient. And it's exactly this level of personal attention that every patient needs.

When we work with a practice, we set up our appointment coordinators in a quiet area away from the hustle and bustle of the office. That way, no matter what they're doing when the phone rings, they're able to answer it with positivity and intentionality. Each phone call is a lifeline to building a lifelong relationship with the patient, and also in establishing that this isn't the same type of dental practice the patient is used to.

One of the ways we break the old filters of how people traditionally listen to the front office staff is by training our appointment coordinators to answer the phone in a specific way. We encourage them to say, "Hello, this is Leslie. Thank you for calling NextLevel Dental. How may I brighten your smile?" For patients who are accustomed to the old model of dentistry, hearing a smiling voice on the other end of the line saying these words comes as quite a shock! It breaks down barriers and clears away the idea of a dental office as a busy, stressful, and chaotic pain chamber. The appointment coordinator has the power of the first impression, and an important role to play in the industry-wide paradigm shift.

Next is the treatment coordinator. These individuals are often perceived as the "money girls" or "money guys" in a practice. For most patients, going into the treatment coordinator's consult room is like going to the principal's office. You feel like you've done something wrong, and unlike your elementary school principal, the treatment coordinator is going to ask for a lot of money to make it right!

In many dental practices, we see patients suddenly getting "too busy" to meet with the treatment coordinator. A last-minute meeting comes up, or they get an emergency call from home. The treatment coordinator asks if they want to schedule their treatment, and they say yes when they really mean no.

Then, the minute they get out the door, they do what I call "the six-month boogie." If you had a camera out in your parking lot, you'd see the patient dancing around as if you'd given them nitrous! The real reason they're dancing, of course, is that they're delighted they didn't really have to commit to anything. They'll call and cancel that appointment without a second thought, because they never really bought the treatment in the first place.

That's why good treatment coordinators are worth their weight in gold. It's your team's job to direct patients toward their office in a positive, upbeat way. It shouldn't be like marching them to the principal's office. On the contrary, the treatment coordinator is there to help. Her job is to help patients fit treatment into their lifestyle so they can look and feel good. She's the one who makes total health and wellness possible. Nobody has a budget for dentistry: it's just not something we budget for. So a treatment coordinator's job is to break down the money barrier for each patient and make total health and wellness financially feasible.

Not only does the treatment coordinator have an important role to play with existing patients; she's also indispensable to retaining the new ones. It's imperative that she be a part of each new patient interview. This gives the patient an opportunity to spend one-on-one time with her, reinforcing that she's not the "money girl"; she's a caring person, their concierge and confidante in being healthy and looking good. She's not their principal; she's their point person for helping them get whatever they need and fitting it into their lifestyle. This interview begins the process of reprogramming a patient's filters.

When people have the opportunity to share in a safe space—not in front of other patients, not in the reception area, not over the counter, but sitting on a comfortable couch in a tastefully decorated room—they feel valued and at ease. They have the opportunity to talk and get to know one another. We teach the treatment coordinator to ask questions like, "What are your past dental experiences? What motivated you to come to us? What are your fears and concerns and issues?" By initiating this dialogue, the treatment coordinator becomes a trusted individual.

When you consider the significance of this new relationship, you'll understand why if you don't currently have a treatment coordinator, you should get one immediately. It's a full-time position. Some dentists tell me they can't bring on a new person because they don't think they'll be getting enough treatment plans to justify it. But when you understand all the dynamics that a quality treatment coordinator brings to the table, you'll see why you can't afford *not* to.

In the new model of dentistry, treatment coordinators aren't money-grubbers, dreaded principals, or a salary sump. On the contrary: they're fundamental members of the care team to get people healthy and well. When they have this strength of purpose, the patient senses it and begins to respect and listen to them on a whole new level.

And that's it. Those are the four key players in a dental office besides the dentist—the dental assistant, hygienist, appointment coordinator, and treatment coordinator. These are the individuals who, through their combined and individual efforts, are transforming the dental office into the epicenter of total health and wellness—a place for patients to be cared for, nurtured, comforted, educated, valued, and supported. It's a place for preemptive and preventative medicine.

The revolution is happening in offices around the country right now. If we can get 100,000 practices to create this paradigm shift in their dental office, we have the potential to impact 300 million people. Imagine how exponentially we can affect the American citizen's healthcare dollar once we reach that level!

Now, if you're reading these pages and you're a dentist, you may feel a little affronted. Perhaps you're thinking, "Hey, *I'm* the doctor. If my team are the ones with all the power, then what am I doing here? I might as well be obsolete!" Far from it, my friend. Dentists in the revolution are not taking on a lesser role; they're simply repositioning themselves. It's your job to empower your team. And here's the good news: it actually frees you up to do more of what you want to do.

I often see dentists trying to wear too many hats. They're sitting chairside and trying to be a business owner at the same time, which necessarily affects the quality of their dentistry. Or they're trying to be an octopus, with their hands in all parts of the practice. But that's not how dentists are the most effective. They have to delegate by putting functioning systems and processes in place. They have to put the right people in the right roles to maximize success.

We just started working with a Pankey/Dawson-trained dentist who's had his practice for thirty years. As a result of our work together, he is beginning to transfer new patients through the hygiene department so that the hygienist can build that crucial relationship. This was, at first, against his traditional training and he was resistant. Now he sees how it saved him an incredible amount of time and made him far more productive. Treatment acceptance is going through the roof because of that one simple change.

The one team position we haven't touched on is the "team leader." The team leader is indispensable to the dentist—they're the one who makes sure you get maximum productivity out of every minute you spend in your practice. The team leader is your new best friend.

In the old model, every dental office had someone called the office manager who moved papers around and processed paperwork. The office manager usually sat in an office on the sidelines. In the new model, we've reinvented this position and reimagined it. The team leader is nothing like the office manager. Team leaders are dynamic, competent, and engaged in the daily inertia of running a practice, from dealing with patients to dealing with the team.

Office managers spend 90 percent of their time putting out fires and 10 percent presenting cases, but we put systems and structures in place so that there are only three things they should be doing—the 3 Ms of management: measuring, monitoring, and making things go right.

Our team leaders are not stuck in a back office in a reactive role like the office managers of yesteryear. They're actually on the court, being proactive. They're supporting and empowering the team, overhearing conversations, correcting the systems and processes that are in place, and then, most importantly, reporting back to the dentist. In our model, the dentist schedules a one-hour meeting with the team leader once a week. During this hour, the team leader is able to share all the pertinent information with the dentist, and then go off and execute all the things that need to be done with the dentist's blessing.

In the new paradigm, dentists only "work" on their practice for an hour a week. They're no longer staying late at the office sorting through paperwork on nights and weekends. This frees the dentist up to have more time to herself.

Our clients use that free time in a number of different ways. Some do speaking engagements at the local community center; others offer free dentistry to people in need. They have time to give back and go out into the world as pioneers of total health and wellness. When people see that the doctor is donating their time, energy, and effort to educate people about dentistry, there's a shift in the paradigm of how they listen.

Every member of your team has an essential role to play as a pioneer of total health and wellness. The better you are able to empower and support them, the more your business will grow, and the faster the revolution will unfold.

Once your team is functioning like a well-oiled machine, it's time to turn your attention to your home life. In the next chapter, we're going to talk about your spouse and your family, and how you can't have a successful dental practice without them.

Chapter 8 — Takeaways

> ❯ Your team members are the key to the dental revolution. Each one has an important role to play.

> ❯ Dental assistants are NJAs: Not Just Assistants. They're the most trusted individuals in a dental office.

> ❯ We can build the power and influence of assistants by helping them view themselves in 3D: Developing Dentistry through Discernment.

> ❯ The hygienist is the second most trusted individual in a dental office, not just the "cleaning lady." Hygienists are the only healthcare practitioners who get two full hours with a patient each year.

> ❯ Hygienists can educate patients on the mouth being the gateway to total health if they simply shift their perspective to 3D: Developing Dentistry through Detection.

> ❯ Appointment coordinators have the power of the first impression; they set the tone for establishing new patient filters. We've expanded their role to 3D: Developing Dentistry through Demeanor.

> ❯ A good treatment coordinator can make case acceptance skyrocket. She's not a "money girl"; she's the patient's concierge and confidante.

❯ Consider hiring or appointing a team leader. They consolidate the work of running a practice and make your life a lot easier.

❯ As a dentist, it's up to you to empower your team. Your team members aren't replacing you. They're freeing you up to do the kind of dentistry you love.

CHAPTER 9

IF YOU AREN'T
HAPPY AT HOME...

FOR MORE THAN SEVENTEEN YEARS, I've watched dentists experience exponential success in their practices as they've applied the principles we teach. These dentists have turned around a system of broken and cancelled appointments, built stellar relationships with new and existing patients, and revolutionized the way people perceive dentistry. The dental revolution is already underway; we see it every day in action. But one thing I've learned is that if you don't have a successful home life, you can't find true success in your practice. Or, if you do, you won't be able to maintain it for long.

Having the support of a partner is crucial, whether it's your husband, wife, girlfriend, or boyfriend. Unfortunately, not every dentist has it. Eighty percent of the dentists we have worked with have been divorced at least once. The issue is complicated by an interesting dynamic unique to dentistry: it's one of the few industries where a high percentage of spouses are actively involved in the work of the practice.

In the traditional model, it's the man who's the dentist. (We'll talk about female dentists and their relationships later in the chapter. Don't worry, ladies—you're not the challenge here!) Of all the dentists I've worked with, only 5 percent have a wife who is completely out of the practice. 60 percent of dentists' wives have an active role in the practice—they're hygienists or assistants or team leaders. Then there are the wives who deal with the practice from home; they handle the bookkeeping or the management side from a distance. They make up 25 percent. The final 10 percent are husband-wife teams where both spouses are dentists in the same practice.

That means that *85 percent of spouses* who aren't dentists themselves are actively involved in their husband's practice. That's a lot!

The number one reason why the wife or significant other works in the practice is because the dentist doesn't do a good job giving them what they need. As I learned from one of my mentors, Martin Cohen, every woman needs four things from her man: financial security, emotional security, love both given and received, and a sense of fun.

I like to think of it this way: your wife or girlfriend needs you to FEEL. She's looking to you for: Fun, Economic security, Emotional security, and Love.

Providing the "EE" of FEEL is the biggest challenge for dentists. Not knowing that their wives need these two types of security, they come home and complain about how there's not enough money coming in, or how the team is failing to live up to their expectations. Faced with this kind of uncertainty, the wife's only recourse is to become actively involved in the practice so that she'll get the assurance she needs.

We expect a lot from our wives. In most families, they're the ones taking care of the home, the kids, and to some extent, the relationship. Because of the culture we live in, women *still* encounter a glass ceiling in the workplace— just compare average wages between the sexes and you'll see it's not an even split. Women are geared to nurture and take care of, but they're also worried about the specifics of survival. This fear can create deep tension in a romantic relationship.

I know this from personal experience. In the past, I used to unload all my financial burdens on my wife, which wasn't fair to her and caused a lot of unnecessary stress in our marriage. Now I channel my complaints and frustrations through my business coach or financial advisor. Sometimes we may have a bad month, but that doesn't give me the right to instill emotional or financial insecurity into my wife's world.

So those are the two Es of FEELing men—Emotional and Economic security. They're the two big ones. We also want to offer Fun and Love to our partners. Women need their husbands to be fun and positive. They also want their man to be able to give and receive love freely. In other words, they want their man to be a good lover, which means being emotionally available. Once you've identified these basic needs, you'll be better able to fulfill them.

Just like there are specific things women need from men, there are also specific things men need from women. Men look to their wives and girlfriends for VISA: Vision, Independence, Safety, and Acknowledgment.

Women are more future-based than we are, and we rely on them to see things that we can't see. I truly consider my wife Judith a visionary. She shows me the way; then I step in and take the lead. It may look like I'm leading, but ultimately, Judith is the one giving me direction and lighting my path! It's like that great line from the movie *My Big Fat Greek Wedding*: the husband may be the head of the family, but the wife is the neck, and she turns the head whichever way she wants!

Men also want their women to be independent. There's nothing more exciting than a woman who knows who she is and what she wants. Then there's the issue of safety, which is the most often misunderstood. Whereas women look to men for financial security, men are seeking a kind of emotional stability from their partners. When a husband senses that his wife is going to turn on an emotional dime at any moment, he feels like he's standing on a median in the middle of a busy highway—no matter which way he turns, he's going to get whacked. A man needs to feel safe in the relationship, able to be and express himself honestly, without retaliation.

The final thing men want from women is acknowledgment and praise. We all want to know that we're doing a good job; that validation is important for us. Our wives are our best cheerleaders, and their support means the world.

Vision, Independence, Safety, and Acknowledgment. Now that's the VISA every wife should carry!

So we've spelled out what men and women need. Wives need husbands who FEEL, and husbands need wives with VISA. Now let's apply it to the context of a dental practice. Ready to put on your helmet and shoulder pads?

That's right—if you want a successful marriage as a dentist, you're going to have to take on a new role: that of champion varsity football player.

Imagine yourself as the prom king and quarterback of the high school football team. What's your job as quarterback? To put on your uniform, go out there, and win games. You're providing security for your teammates by putting points on the board. It's your responsibility to be the team leader. When you play your role correctly, you're providing security for everyone—your team on the field, your fans in the stands, and the cheerleaders on the sidelines. Why does the whole stadium erupt into cheers when you toss that 40-yard touchdown pass? Because they feel secure!

If you're the prom king quarterback, then your wife's the prom queen and head cheerleader. She's rooting for you out on the field. If you make a bad play, she's not going to scowl at you and sit on her pom-poms. She's going to get right back in there to encourage and support you. Even if you make a mistake, she's there to say, "Hey, don't worry! We're going to get 'em anyway." She's providing the future vision and the acknowledgment you need.

It's a metaphor, but it's a powerful one. These roles are exactly the roles husbands and wives should be playing in their marriages! The dentist is the captain of the team in the dental office—he's the play-maker, the guy in charge. He's the one scoring victories with patients and providing support and security for his team. That sense of leadership carries over at home, where he provides financial and emotional security for his wife. Meanwhile, she's providing him with the validation, praise, and vision he needs to succeed.

What does the quarterback do? He wins games. And what does a cheerleader do? She never quits on her quarterback. She never stops cheering for her team. If you run your marriage like the big game, then everybody's happy!

Of course, as I've experienced, most dentists don't approach their marriages this way—at least not their first marriages. The reason divorce rates among male dentists are so high is because, not knowing that these are the things husbands and wives need from each other, they keep pushing all the wrong buttons. The tension escalates as neither partner is satisfied. You can reverse the downward spiral by understanding what each person needs and communicating from that perspective. But if you stay mired in past failures, you won't be able to move forward, and since most dentists are on their second marriages, their past failures are often particularly vibrant in their minds.

We teach dental team members to see every patient in a new light each time they come in. The same is true for your spouse. Every day with your spouse is a new day; both of you are changing, learning, and growing. Every day I wake up next to my wife, I look at her as a new woman, full of new insight and wisdom. If I don't blank-slate my relationship every day, then I carry the past into the present and Judith never gets the opportunity to be who she is in the moment because I've smothered her by my past beliefs. Of course, don't *really* go find a new woman to wake up to every day. If you're tempted to, just remember that the grass isn't greener on the other side; it's greener where you water it and shine light on it!

When we work with clients who have been divorced, we urge them to take responsibility for their part in the failure of a past relationship. It's never a one-way street. We do exercises to help them work backward and figure out what didn't work about their former marriage or relationship, and what role they played.

Then, instead of carrying old baggage into a new relationship, we have them draw a line in the sand. We help them bring closure to the past. That frees them up to acknowledge what is working with their current partner and what isn't. Instead of playing the blame game, they take responsibility for their own role. And once they talk it out with their partner, they can come to an agreement going forward on what each of them needs in the relationship.

In our workshops and live events, I ask dentists: Why did you get married? What made you first fall in love with your partner? By remembering why they got married in the first place, the dentist is able to recall the common values he and his wife once shared. It's easy for those values to get clouded over when life gets in the way—by heartbreak, difficulty, and even simply the passage of time. But reconnecting to those common values can help you survive the circumstantial breakdowns in communication that will inevitably arise.

As parents of a child diagnosed with autism, my wife and I have had our share of hardships. There's a fundamental lack of communication that happens with children diagnosed with autism, and substantial financial drain. Sound familiar? That's because it is! In many ways, Judith and I face the same challenges a dentist does. Eighty-five percent of parents of children with autism are divorced, which isn't far removed from the 80 percent of dentists who've had broken marriages. There are so many pressures and challenges to contend with, and sometimes it can feel like they're hitting you from all sides.

But there's hope. Judith and I continue to strengthen our relationship by finding ways to be there for our son, *and* for each other. For us, that means taking our relationship to the next level and having it stand for something bigger than just ourselves. The three things everyone wants to experience in their partnership are fun, love, and making a difference. When it comes to that last one, it's about standing for something purposeful in the world.

For my wife, it's helping parents of kids with autism. For me, it's helping people be happy, healthy, and well in dentistry. Judith and I come together and have conversations about our greater purpose—about using our partnership to leave a legacy. Every day, we focus on moving beyond just being quarterback and cheerleader to each other, and being leaders and team players for the rest of the world.

With dentists, the opportunities are exciting. What happens when you break out of the stadium and start bringing the joy and transformation to the fans? I'm seeing it now with dentists who are pioneering the dental revolution. Once their marriage is secure, they're able to secure their practice, and once their practice is working, they go out into their communities to share what they've learned. When you're no longer bogged down by the stresses and heartache of a conflicted relationship, you can shift to a whole new level with your partner and channel your combined efforts into leaving a legacy.

When both partners are empowered to do work that is meaningful to them, dependency issues within a relationship begin to dissolve. The male dentist is able to get clear on his own vision for the practice without always having to rely on his wife to play visionary. Many women decide that their time is best spent *outside* of the practice. So they step out and find their own position in the world, making a life for themselves as independent women.

I'm not saying that wives shouldn't be involved in their husband's dental practice. Far from it—it can be a wonderful thing. But it's important that every dentist *find his voice*. They're telling their patients to "open wide," but they're not opening wide themselves. And in reality, it's often not the wife who is dependent on her husband; it's the husband who's dependent on the wife!

Recently, after working with a male client, we received a letter from his wife. "I'm so proud of my husband!" she said. "He's taking charge and really doing great. Thank you for empowering him and I!" What had happened was that she stepped out of the practice and finally gave him the space to find his voice.

One of the things dentists struggle with most is confrontation. A lot of them just don't want to confront difficult situations, so they either get their wife to do it or hire a practice consultant. We teach our clients how to confront issues on their own—and that means at home, too. If you don't have the muscle for confrontation with your wife, then you won't develop it with your team, and if you don't develop it with your team, then you won't be able to present treatment to your patients.

Our goal is to give dentists the tools they need to have hard conversations. As a result, they're able to strengthen their communication skills and really find their voices. Once they've gotten better at talking to their wives, team members, and patients, it's only natural that they begin talking to their colleagues and the greater public. They can say what they need to say to all the people in their lives, and they're able to give back to their family, their community, and the great industry we've all been privileged to work in.

As you've probably surmised by now, most female dentists don't face the same set of problems. When I ask a woman to tell me her vision, she has no trouble articulating exactly what she wants and how she plans to get there. But when I ask a male dentist the same question, it's like pulling teeth!

Ten percent of female dentists work alongside their dentist husbands. The other statistics vary considerably. Only 20 percent of female dentists' husbands are actively involved in the practice, and another 20 percent are involved from home. A whopping 50 percent aren't involved at all!

To the female dentist, all I have to say is: You've got it going on. Your relationships with your partners are a model for the rest of us!

For the rest of us, it's never too late to turn things around. Your wife is always going to be the head cheerleader. You're always going to be the quarterback. Think of every day as the big game, and every night as prom night...for the rest of your life. Once you've established the security and safety you need in your home life, you'll be ready to tackle the rest of the world.

In Chapter 10, get ready to step up. The new vision of dentistry is here, and it's yours for the taking.

Chapter 9 — Takeaways

> ❯ To achieve success in your practice, you must first establish a healthy relationship with your partner at home.

> ❯ Women like men who FEEL. They need husbands and boyfriends who can provide Fun, Economic security, Emotional security, and Love.

> ❯ Men need women who can offer them VISA: Vision, Independence, Safety, and Acknowledgment.

> ❯ In your marriage or relationship, think of yourself as the high school quarterback and your significant other as head cheerleader. Every day of your marriage should be prom night!

> ❯ Make a point not to drag past baggage into your current relationship. Instead, treat every day as a new day, and treat your partner as a fresh, new human being.

> ❯ It's important that you *find your voice*. Use it to create and clarify the vision of your dental practice, and to confront issues on your own.

> ❯ Once you and your partner are secure in your relationship to each other and your children, turn your attention outward to your greater purpose. How can you leave a legacy for the world?

CHAPTER 10

A NEW VISION: DENTISTRY DELIVERS HEALTH AND WELLNESS

DENTISTS WHO HAVE COMPLETED one of our programs often tell me the same thing. "My life has gotten dramatically better," they say. "And the main thing that changed was me."

That's just it. What we've been talking about in this book doesn't require you to make some cataclysmic change. It's not about doing more things or working more hours. It's about a fundamental transformation that happens *within* you and then spreads to every single area of your life.

We're talking about dental revolution. And the revolution begins *inside of you.*

This book has been about changing your relationship to the people and things in your life. It starts with your relationship to yourself, and the realization that suffering is *not* mandatory—that it's optional. This new understanding soon spreads to your home life, strengthening your relationships with your spouse and your children. Then it moves to the relationships you have with your team members and the patients in your practice, and your relationships to time and money. And finally, it expands to include your relationships with your colleagues, your community, and the industry of dentistry itself.

This is the key to dental revolution. We're not just talking about a paradigm shift in dentistry. We're talking about a paradigm shift in every relationship that defines your world.

It's easy to read a book like this and say, "It all sounds great. But this isn't for me—it's for the other guy. The one with charisma and the great life."

I'm here to tell you: this isn't for the other guy. It's for you.

Maybe you don't see yourself as a pioneer of the dental revolution. Maybe you're more of a frontier person or a settler. Wherever you are, that's okay. We'll meet you there.

And if the idea of revolution still scares you, don't let it. It's not about investing more time or money or energy; it's about re-prioritizing the things you *are* doing. It's about shifting your relationships and your perspective. That shift creates an opening, and when the time is right, you'll be able to step into that void.

"How do I step into that void?" you ask. "What would my life look like if I were to move into that open space?"

The answer is: You'll give back all that's been given to you.

Now we've come full circle. We started on a journey that was deeply personal; in the next phase, it expanded to include your dental practice; now, in the final phase, we are reaching even further outward. It's about being of service, about giving back to your industry, your community, and healthcare itself. It's about leaving a legacy that's going to make a lasting difference in the world.

As we stand on the precipice of a massive healthcare overhaul and a complete overturning of the medical establishment as we know it, I see limitless potential. I see a system being turned on its head, and in that chaos, I see the opportunity for dentists to rise up, join together, and give the world what it is aching for: total health and wellness, administered by caring and competent healthcare practitioners. The economist Joseph Schumpeter many years ago coined the term "creative destruction." It's what happens in the economy when one order collapses and a new one rises to take its place.

In this book, I've laid out a vision for you. It's a brand new vision, one the world has never seen, but that the world desperately needs. It's a vision of dentistry delivering medicine, but beyond that, delivering total health and wellness to millions of people around the country.

I urge you to step up and fill the gap that has been created by fluctuating healthcare policies and system-wide changes. This is your opportunity to shine. It is your moment to become the primary provider in American healthcare—the vanguard of the revolution. You have a new story to tell, a new way to approach dentistry, a new song to sing. You no longer have to keep your head down. Everything in your life is about to get radically better, starting with you and ending farther than the eye can see—as far as you can imagine. You can have it all.

"Having it all" isn't about what you can take from the world, but what you can give to it. The dental revolution I have described in these pages is about being *of* service. If you have a great life, you're more inclined to share it—not just with the people in your family and on your team, but with the world at large.

That's why we created *learning centers*. The concept of a learning center is that it allows dentists to act as mutual mentors to other dental teams, guiding them along their own walk to reach this final level of personal and professional evolution. When you begin to experience unprecedented success, it's the most natural thing in the world to want to share it with others. There is more than enough—enough patients, enough money, enough success—for everyone.

In Chapter 9, we talked about dentists finding their voices inside their practices. Once you've done so, it's time to find your voice *outside* your practice. Everything you know about dentistry, everything that's different about the new model, must be shouted from the rooftops. It's up to you to spread the word.

And you're already doing it. The positive messaging is beginning to take hold—in conversations people are having with one another, in the news. I see it everywhere I look. Oral health has captivated the public mind. It's showing up on *The Today Show with Matt Lauer*, in *Newsweek*, on Dr. Oz's top ten list of tips for living a long life. Bit by bit, dentistry is getting a media makeover, and people are beginning to listen through different filters.

Yes, some negative messaging persists. As I mentioned earlier, I recently heard an ad on the radio that said, "Getting a mortgage doesn't have to be as painful as going to the dentist!" But every day I see people in our noble industry combating those negative messages. Step by step, we're turning our image around.

It's not a one-man or a one-woman job. It's going to take a big group of men and women going out into the world and reeducating the public. It's up to us to take a stand for the new model of dentistry, to reposition dentists as the primary healthcare provider of total health and wellness.

It's time to stop hiding from the truth, and the truth is that you have made and continue to make a profound difference in the lives of many. Now that you know that, now that your team knows that, now that your patients know that, it's time to give it away to other practitioners—to let them know that the same thing is possible for them.

This is a defining moment. Because of the shifts and jolts in our world, there is going to be a new normal. We've essentially ruined the medical system, and if someone doesn't step up to the plate, we're looking at many years of ineffective care and mass suffering with no end in sight.

The dentist is the next great American hero. It's up to you to step in and lead the charge.

It's not just up to you. It's up to everybody who is connected to dentistry. It's up to every team leader, every assistant, every hygienist, every treatment coordinator, every appointment coordinator. It's up to the loyal partners and spouses working behind the scenes. It's up to the Invisalign territory managers and Henry Schein reps, and the executives and board members of major dental companies. If we collectively get together and combine forces across our vast industry, imagine the scope of our potential. Imagine the kind of legacy we could leave.

It's easy to become mired in day-to-day complaints—the seemingly never-ending process of running a practice—but there is a life beyond where you are now. While it may seem like a huge mountain to climb, all you have to do is take the first step. Once you take that first step, you gain momentum, and it doesn't have to stop. In fact, on the contrary, it will continue to build and grow.

I've struggled through my own periods of doubt. There have been times when it seemed easier to give up, to throw in the towel and say, "What am I talking about, dental revolution? It's crazy!" But I have a vision for what is possible, and that vision has allowed me to keep forging through the many highs and lows. There is nothing more powerful in life than standing for something bigger than yourself.

Can you imagine the difference we could make to people's health? Can you envision the contribution we could make to the world?

I can. It's time to make that vision a reality.

We may have reached the end of this book, but it's also a new beginning. The journey has just begun. The time is now.

My final words to you?

The future is yours. The future is *ours.*

In the words of one of my favorite client's son, Andrew, "The tragedy in life is that it is not too short; the tragedy in life is that it takes too darn long to get going."

Go ahead. Giddyup. Get going. Now!

Chapter 10 — Takeaways

> The dental revolution doesn't start "out there." It starts with you, in the transformation in your relationships to the people and things in your world.

> The revolution isn't for "the other guy." It's for you.

> If we join forces, we can not only create a paradigm shift in dentistry, but in the entire American healthcare system.

> The time to act is now. Let's get going!